Integrative Imaging in Neuroplasticity, Wisdom and Neuropsychiatry

Science Meets Arts (SMART)

By

Yongxia Zhou

Integrative Imaging in Neuroplasticity, Wisdom and Neuropsychiatry: Science Meets Arts (SMART)

By Yongxia Zhou

This book first published 2023

Ethics International Press Ltd, UK

British Library Cataloguing in Publication Data

A catalogue record for this book is available from the British Library

Print Book ISBN: 978-1-80441-358-6

eBook ISBN: 978-1-80441-104-9

TABLE OF CONTENTS

Preface

Neuroimaging of chess players such as grand masters and comparison to matched controls might help reveal the neuroplasticity changes in brain such as cognition and problem solving abilities. Neural underpins of behavioral data could further elucidate the neurobiological connections and the underlying neural mechanism due to training effects, especially for long-term professional practice. Also brain science including topics of cognitive function such as music/creativity training and experience as well as scientific education including mathematical calculation, learning and memory could be investigated with neuroimaging approaches that provide objective and *in vivo* imaging evidence of specific brain functional and structural neuronal resources utilization and relocation. For instance, music experience such as singing, listening, playing and professional improvisation activated several brain circuits including emotion regulation such as relief and pleasure, reward perception from anticipation to consumption, language system such as comprehension and communication as well as motor function from planning to coordination. Furthermore, for well education, college life cultivates professional skills, improves social interaction and communication, broadens vision and expands mind, gains experience and expertise and finally enriches knowledge and creativity. Emotional intelligence (EI) and general intelligence that were used for reasoning and analyzing to solve problems are usually emphasized for improvement during academic training. People with normal and high intelligence, especially superior EI ability, could perform better in complicate environment and obtain more academic achievement with successful appraisal, monitoring, utilization of emotions and social skills. Also positive effects of emotional regulation and facilitation in after-college life had showed promotions of creativity and mood in better working environment as well as enhanced interpersonal communication with better EI. Finally, watching movie paradigm with fMRI could be used to improve brain function and characterize individual variation due to different art contents, culture, background and environment. Several issues had been addressed such as session and condition differences due to the specific length and focused smooth activation patterns of movie fMRI, for the applications in neuroscience and neuropsychiatry. The beneficial effects in brain circuits involving memory and attention, reward and social values, decision making and coordination, creativity and persistence of these skills as well as expertise including chess practice, music/counting training, college education and watching-picture/movie were reviewed and investigated with full-spectrum, solid and up-to-date experimental data utilizing advanced quantitative imaging techniques in the first four chapters of this book. Associated phenotypic correlations were further illustrated to validate the training and learning imaging evidence together with anticipated neuroprotective and neurodevelopmental improvements with multiple neuroimaging modalities.

Attention-deficit and hyperactivity disorder (ADHD) is a relatively high prevalent neurodevelopmental disease, having about 6% prevalence rate worldwide. It had been reported that age and family socioeconomic status affected the prevalence of ADHD in children and adolescents, with more comorbid symptoms such as additional loss of impulsivity in adults. ADHD could be classified into the primary combined and inattentive subtypes from the typically-developed (TD) controls. Neuroimaging findings included both intra- and inter- network hyper-connectivities in ADHD group compared to TD controls, such as abnormally increased connectivities from typical functional default mode network (DMN), central executive network (CEN), salience and visual networks. Furthermore, numerous studies have been performed to investigate brain changes associated with drug addiction for better treatment and recovery effects. As another example, inverse coupling between DMN and CEN was increased after nicotine replacement pharmacotherapy, and these inter- and intra-network changes including enhanced CEN and reward systems were related to the withdrawal symptom improvement. And in the substance-dependent brain, large-scale network communication efficiency was lower via small-worldness analysis with disruption of inter-regional regulation topology, indicating possible loss of inhibition and addiction risk of drug seeking behavior. The second part of this book illustrated specific brain functional and structural changes of ADHD and drug dependence in chapters 5 and 6. In addition to multiparametric and novel imaging analysis and applications in real and relatively new database, integrative neuroscientific findings and therapeutic evaluation with neuroimaging techniques were also reviewed.

Comprehensive imaging investigation of the arts and science training effects in professionals, early college learning experience, daily skills and culture-based practice on brain were thoroughly exhibited in this new book. Expected improvements and novel functional/structural gains of brain regions and circuits in several aspects including reward/emotion/intelligence/decision making were emphasized and detailed. Brain reserve, especially the neuroplasticity and wisdom accumulation over lifetime education and intellectual activities/experience could preserve healthy cognitive-emotional structure, remain less vulnerable to functional impairments and protect against neuropsychiatric disease challenges. The aim of this new book is thus intended to provide both beginners and experts in biomedical imaging and general public health a broad and complete brain picture of positive arts and science training benefits with thorough analysis and solid data covering college education to professional expertise. Extensive applications in common diseases together with the cutting-edge and full-spectrum static and dynamic, functional and structural, regional and inter-network, imaging and phenotypic characteristics are the highlights and advantage of this book. We would hope to capture the interests of colleagues and researchers in the areas of neuroplasticity imaging, neurodevelopmental and neuropsychiatric applications as well as disease diagnosis and treatment. The ultimate goal is to convey the methodological innovation and neuroscientific applications of important education, health, arts and science-related topics. The author would also like to acknowledge the open NeuroImaging Tools & Resources Collaboratory (NITRC) database for sharing and managing the original imaging data, and especially the precious resources provided by several Chinese research branches in Chapters 1, 3 and 5.

Chapter 1 – Imaging evidence of brain cognitive and neuroplasticity changes associated with chess practicing skills and expertise had been reported. In this study, we found consistent gray matter density and interhemispheric correlation changes in chess players compared to controls, including both higher in the superior frontal, medial prefrontal cortex and visual/cerebellum regions. The VMHC identified extra hypo-connectivity in the parietal and cuneus regions but hyper-conductivity in the temporal cortex and subcortical basal ganglia and hypothalamus, while VBM localized further higher gray matter densities in the orbitofrontal, caudate, cuneus and supplementary motor areas in the chess group. These primarily increased gray matter densities and connectivity in critical brain regions indicated expected improvement of cognitive function including decision planning and making (supplementary motor and superior frontal), memory and attention (posterior temporal and orbitofrontal), visuospatial ability (occipital) and movement coordination (subcortical and cerebellum) in chess masters. In line with the structural/conductivity changes, increased intra- and inter-network connectivities of several crucial brain networks were identified, including visual network (VN), central executive network (CEN), thalamocortical circuits such as motor network (MN), default mode network (DMN)-medial frontal region, frontoparietal network (FPN) as well as the salience network (SN) in the chess players compared to controls. Increased dynamic correlations of typical brain networks such as VN, CEN, MN and DMN/CEN together with longer dwell time/occupancy/frequency for optimal strategy in chess players had also been confirmed. Moreover, global neural activity and regional synchrony signals were enhanced in chess professionals compared to controls, together with the higher absolute local efficiency for faster local neural source utilization.

Multiple brain activity/connectivity and phenotypic data had been revealed in chess group mostly. For instance, associations were observed between Raven's RPM score and neural activity in the superior frontal and posterior cingulate region as well as between Raven's score and gray matter density in the temporal and occipital clusters. Professional rate correlated positively with cerebellar regional synchrony, while starting age was negatively related to the interhemispheric conductivity in the salience network and temporal/cuneus region. Some other correlations existed such as positive correlations between levels and frontal VMHC, between start age and subcortical ReHo/fALFF, possibly due to neuroprotective and compensatory mechanisms. Finally, consistent whole-brain voxel-wise and regional tract-specific DTI FA increments were present in chess group, including the arcuate fasciculus, inferior longitudinal and inferior fronto-occipital fascicle, corpus callosum and cortico-spinal tract. Tight links between DTI FA together with diffusivity (AD/RD/MD) metrics and phenotypic data were discovered as well, including between bilateral inferior longitudinal fasciculus/cingulum diffusivity/FA and training time/professional level in chess group. Our comprehensive results complemented previous findings, validating the multi-level (static and dynamic, local and global, structural and functional) brain quantitative gains in chess training and cognitive practice.

Chapter 2 – In this work, we had performed all six conditional VMHC comparisons, including each of three task conditions vs. resting state, as well as between two-task comparisons. Similar brain patterns of lower VMHC in the visual, temporal and somatosensory, motor areas in music/counting/memory conditions compared to resting state were observed. Between-comparisons for each two of three tasks further demonstrated the distinct regional allocation of neural resources under three conditions, including medial prefrontal, anterior cingulate, insular, superior temporal, occipital, thalamus, cerebellum and motor/supplementary motor areas related to music singing condition, with more differences comparing music to counting than memory conditions. The counting condition revealed more orbitofrontal interhemispheric correlation in addition to specific intra-parietal sulcus (IPS) and superior frontal gyrus (SFG) conductivity compared to music/memory. While clusters in the medial temporal lobe including hippocampus and parahippocampus, posterior cingulate, precuneus, dorsolateral prefrontal cortex (DLPFC) and superior parietal lobe maintained higher VMHC during episodic memory recall processing than music and counting tasks.

Functional connectivity based ICA-DR algorithm identified enhanced network connectivities of intra- DMN, FPN and SN during music singing condition compared to counting and memory recall tasks. On the other hand, lower inter-network connectivities including inter- DMN and FPN, frontal and temporal network (FTN) were observed due to possible neural source shifting and deactivation. Higher intra- and inter- FPN, VN, FTN, VN-DMN and

SN network connectivities in counting condition compared to music and memory tasks were discovered, consistent with the hyper-connectivity of IPS/SFG/DLPFC VMHC values. Finally, as expected, more connection of intra- and inter- temporal, DMN-FPN, FTN and thalamo-cortical circuit were present during episodic memory recall condition. The dFNC connectogram confirmed the higher temporal dynamics of six representative networks such as higher DMN-CEN-MN connections at three task conditions compared to resting state. Small-worldness analysis revealed slightly higher global but lower local efficiencies in counting and music conditions together with relatively higher small-worldness weighting factor in the memory condition compared to resting state. Our multimodal neuroimaging results were consistent with published findings for each separate condition, and provided extra imaging evidence of arts and science training-related neuroplasticity and dynamic modulation enhancement in brain structure and function.

Chapter 3 – The objectives of this chapter were to investigate the brain changes such as neural activity and myelin-related functional correlation as well as morphological/microstructural connectivity-based neuroplasticity improvements during college training with baseline and longitudinal imaging and phenotypic data. For the fALFF correlational results, several regions presented significantly positive correlations between fALFF neural activities and four aspects of emotional intelligence (EI) scores including insula, hypothalamus, cuneus and motor areas at all three time points. Longitudinally, increased associations between fALFF and EI scores were observed in the visuospatial regions and frontal medial/dorso-lateral portions. For trait association, fALFF neural activities in some similar regions such as frontal, motor/supplementary motor areas, thalamus, basal ganglia and temporoparietal regions also presented negative association with different aspects of the trait scores at three time points. For the ReHo associations, EI scores including all four aspects were positively associated with regional homogeneity in the parietal/superior temporal cluster and premotor/motor areas. During all the three time points, Raven's CRT score was positively associated with ReHo values in the orbitofrontal and superior frontal, insular, superior temporal and motor/supplementary motor areas. For the VMHC, significant longitudinal increments in the inferior temporal area, posterior cingulate and inferior parietal regions were observed. VMHC values in the cerebellum, temporal cortex including hippocampus/parahippocampus and superior segment, sensorimotor area and occipital/parietal lobes showed consistently negative associations with the depression/anxiety scores.

Significant positive correlations between gray matter density in the cerebellum, insular, orbitofrontal, fusiform, cuneus, posterior cingulate, medial prefrontal, subcortical caudate and putamen regions were observed with the EI scores of four domains including appraisal, monitoring, social ability and utilization at three time points. While cortical temporal regions including hippocampus and parahippocampus, orbitofrontal and superior frontal, visual and sensorimotor areas demonstrated significant correlations and predictions with depression and trait/state anxiety scores mainly. Associations between EI/trait scores and DTI FA/diffusivities in several tracts of the thalamic radiation, splenium of corpus callosum, internal capsule, cingulum, superior longitudinal fasciculus and cortico-spinal tract were identified at all time points. Finally, significantly increased global and decreased local efficiencies longitudinally were identified, indicating a more optimal and efficient brain network topology at later time point after college training. In line with the results presented in previous Chapters 1 and 2, these brain regions showed improvements of neural activity, synchrony and integration, myelin-related conductivity, morphological and microstructural connectivity for better performance and achievement with skills training, emotional and social interaction as well as knowledge accumulation.

Chapter 4 – The purpose of this chapter was to investigate both longitudinal session and conditional effects of fMRI paradigm including movie and flankers stimulation on brain, as well as the associated phenotypical correlations. With ICA-DR algorithm, both session and conditional effects were observed. For instance, during movie-watching, session-differences were reflected in the regions of medial orbitofrontal cortex, medial and superior frontal, middle temporal gyrus, inferior parietal lobe, angular gyrus, motor/premotor area and several regions in the visual cortex including subregions V1-V5, precuneus, cuneus, lingual, intracalcarine and occipital pole. Conditional network-based connectivity alterations such as movie vs. resting and inscape vs. resting comparisons involved mostly precuneus and inferior parietal gyrus. These dynamic network-based correlational changes indicated significant and specific visuo-motion enhancement of emotion/creativity/social communications related to the movie contents and brain cognitive processing. Significant functional network topological property with increased local and global network efficiencies (absolute) at later compared to earlier sessions for all conditions including movie and resting state were identified.

Significantly higher global VMHC Z-value during inscape stimulation compared to rest (P=0.02) and movie conditions (P=0.01) were observed. Global functional activity/conductivity z-value variations of each condition and session were exhibited additionally, such as relatively higher movie/inscape fALFF neural activity compared to rest/flankers conditions. Phenotypic associations were also revealed with fMRI metrics, including positive correlation between fALFF during movie watching condition and internal-state of hunger score as well as negative correlation between fALFF/VMHC global z-values during inscape stimulus and internal hunger/full scores. With dFNC connectogram analysis, similar distribution of mean dwell time of all six states in several sessions were observed with significantly lower mean dwell time in later session compared to baseline. Consistent with previous findings, our quantitative and multiparametric imaging results remained relatively consistent for different types of visual stimulations and tasks, suggesting temporal or long-term neuroplasticity and brain connectogram improvement from artistic and training paradigm such as movie and flankers.

Chapter 5 – The purposes of this chapter were to investigate further brain structural and functional changes in Attention-deficit and hyperactivity disorder (ADHD) combined (AC) and inattention (AI) subtypes compared to typically developed (TD) children with available structural and functional MRI data using multiple advanced imaging methods. For both structural gray matter density (GMD) and interhemispheric correlation, AC group presented significantly larger GMD and VMHC values compared to TD and AI, and relatively close values between AI and TD were found. Specifically, medial orbitofrontal cortex, temporal pole, anterior cingulate, cuneus and supplementary motor area presented both higher values of GDM and VMHC in AC group that might be related to the hyperactivity and attentional deficits in ADHD. Small clusters in the cerebellum, temporal and dorsolateral regions also showed atrophy in AI group compared to TD.

For functional connectivity differences with ICA-DR algorithm, reduced intra- and inter-network connectivities of posterior DMN, visuo-temporal, thalamic-occipital and fronto-temporal networks were observed in AC group compared to TD and AI. However, increased network connectivities in the visual, frontal, anterior DMN, thalamo-temporal, and anterior cingulate-FPN regions were found in AC group. Both relative local efficiency and small-worldness weighting factor were lowest in the AC group but highest

in the AI group, while the absolute local and global efficiencies were abnormally highest in AC but lowest in AI group. Based on dFNC analysis, reversal dFNC connectogram patterns for most states were revealed in AC compared to TD. The mean dwell time was lower in AC compared to TD, and was significantly lower in the AI patients compared to TD group. Our quantitative multiparametric imaging results showed reliable and rigorous brain changes in ADHD and subtypes compared to TD controls.

Chapter 6 – The purposes of this chapter were to identify brain neural correlates of clinical data including drug dependence, with advanced multiparametric imaging quantification including fALFF/ReHo/VMHC, ICA-DR and dFNC. Significant negative associations between functional imaging including fALFF/ ReHo/VMHC as well as intra-/inter- network functional connectivities identified with ICA-DR algorithms with phenotypic data such as dependence and time of use were identified in multiple brain regions, including the ventral striatum, insula, cerebellum, temporal cortex and orbitofrontal cortex together with hypothalamus and ventromedial prefrontal cortex. Education and handcraft experience showed some neuroprotection effects in several regions including the orbitofrontal, ventral striatum, hypothalamus, superior frontal and temporal amygdala/ hippocampus areas. Graph-theory based centrality showed significant correlations between binarized/weighted centrality degree and number of cigarettes per day as well as between weighted local functional connectivity degree centrality and number of cigarettes. Based on dFNC analysis, abnormally hyper-connectivities of connectograms in several states were identified including abnormally higher between-network dynamic correlations (close to 1) of state S4 for all the connections. The number of occurrence was relatively evenly distributed with close to mean value of 16% for all states (similar to the chess control group

as in Chapter 1), while the distribution patterns of frequency and dwell time were similar to those of ADHD-AC type as illustrated in Chapter 5. Therapeutic strategies that target strengthening typical brain circuits in addiction such as CEN, DMN, SN and FPN/MN as well as thalamo-cortical connections might be effective for better brain inter-network modulation and dynamic facilitations with more regular behavior and better emotion/cognitive control.

Chapter 1
Comprehensive Imaging Findings
in Professional Chess Players

Abstract

Imaging evidence of brain cognitive and neuroplasticity changes associated with chess practicing skills and expertise had been reported recently. In this study, we found consistent gray matter density and interhemispheric correlation changes in chess players compared to controls, including both higher in the superior frontal and medial prefrontal cortices as well as visual/cerebellum regions. The VMHC identified extra hypo-connectivity in the parietal and cuneus regions but hyper-conductivity in the temporal cortex and subcortical basal ganglia and hypothalamus, while VBM localized further higher gray matter densities in the orbitofrontal, caudate, cuneus and supplementary motor areas in the chess group. These primarily increased gray matter densities and connectivity in critical brain regions indicated expected improvement of cognitive function including decision planning and making (supplementary motor and superior frontal), memory and attention (posterior temporal and orbitofrontal), visuospatial ability (occipital) and movement coordination (subcortical and cerebellum) in chess masters. In line with the structural/conductivity changes, increased intra- and inter-network connectivities of several crucial brain networks were identified, including visual network (VN), central executive network (CEN), thalamocortical circuits such as motor network (MN), default mode network (DMN)-medial frontal region, frontoparietal network (FPN) as well as the salience network (SN) in the chess players compared to controls. Increased dynamic correlations of typical brain networks such as VN, MN and DMN/CEN together with longer dwell time/occupancy/frequency for optimal strategy in chess players had also been confirmed. Moreover, global neural activity and regional synchrony signals were enhanced in chess professionals compared to controls, together with the higher absolute local efficiency for faster local neural source utilization.

Multiple links between brain activity/connectivity and phenotypic data had been revealed in chess group additionally. For instance, associations were observed between Raven's RPM score and neural activity in the superior frontal and posterior cingulate region as well as between Raven's score and gray matter density in the temporal and occipital clusters. Professional rate correlated positively with cerebellar regional synchrony, while starting age was negatively related to the interhemispheric conductivity in the salience network and temporal/cuneus region. Some other correlations existed such as positive connections between levels and frontal VMHC, between start age and subcortical ReHo/fALFF, possibly due to neuroprotective and compensatory mechanisms. Finally, consistent whole-brain voxel-wise and regional tract-specific DTI FA increments were present in chess group, including the arcuate fasciculus, inferior longitudinal and fronto-occipital fascicle, corpus callosum and cortico-spinal tract. Tight links between DTI FA together with diffusivity (AD/RD/MD) metrics and phenotypic data were discovered as well, including between bilateral inferior longitudinal fasciculus/cingulum diffusivity/FA and training time/professional level in chess group. Our comprehensive results complemented previous findings, validating the multi-level (static and dynamic, local and global, structural and functional) brain quantitative gains in chess training and cognitive practice.

Keywords: fMRI, chess, neuroimaging, functional connectivity, dynamic functional network correlation, functional activity, regional homogeneity, neuroplasticity, intelligence, Raven's progressive matrices score, training effects, gray matter density, interhemispheric correlation, structural connectivity, fractional anisotropy, diffusivity, attention, memory, decision making, movement coordination

1. Introduction

1.1. Overview

Chess is a board game that has long history with significant learning, training, reward and wisdom benefits in China and also the whole world. Neuroimaging of chess players including grand masters and comparison to matched controls might help reveal the neuroplasticity changes in brain such as cognition and problem solving abilities. Neural underpins of behavioral data could further elucidate the neurobiological connections and the underlying neural mechanism due to training effects, especially for long-term professional practice [1]. Based on MRI diffusion tensor imaging (DTI), increased microstructural connectivity and integrity were found in chess players, including inferior longitudinal fasciculus (ILF), superior longitudinal fasciculus (SLF), uncinate fasciculus (UF) and cingulum that had important language and memory function [2]. Also DTI diffusivity in the SLF was negatively associated with chess tournament ranking, and fractional anisotropy (FA) in several tracts including UF and ILF were correlated with Raven's progressive matrices (RPM) score for measuring fluid intelligence [2, 3]. Furthermore, better players with higher intelligence also had more efficient brain functioning, and manifested as higher event-related synchronization of cortical neural activation [4]. Superior chess skills correlated with larger memory capacity of knowledge and patterns based on memory performance tests [5].

Long-term professional training of chess playing emphasizes winning the board game with the shortest time and optimal strategy from complicate and variable dynamic patterns exchanged between two players. The improvements of visuospatial attention and contexture recognition in chess experts had been reported in several studies. For instance, salience and ventral attention networks were anatomically and functionally altered in chess masters compared to amateur players based on brain connectome [6]. Chinese chess experts were found to have thinner cortical depth (a global communication distance measure through anatomical mantle) in several brain regions for visual attention and memory, but with increased functional connectivity to distant brain regions in comparison to novices [7]. These brain changes might indicate chess experts recruited more of these regions for maximizing visuospatial information and exceptional performance [7]. Activity in the brain pattern recognition regions such as posterior temporal and left inferior parietal areas were related to the performance outcome of experts [8]. Enhanced fusiform area activation was reported in experts compared to novices in response to naturalistic full-board chess positions [9]. Finally, the collateral sulci (medial occipitotemporal) on both sides were involved in chess-specific pattern recognition while the occipitotemporal junction was linked to general object recognition in chess experts [8, 10].

Chess expertise practice sharpens long-term memory chunk to allow for quick pattern retrieval and recognition (especially at "win" situation), and these chunks were found to be located primarily in the temporal lobe together with the short-time working memory allocated in the frontal and parietal lobes [11]. Memory tests identified extensive brain activation in the frontal (e.g., medial and inferior segments) and posterior cingulate cortices as well as cerebellum in chess players [12]. In addition, left-sided temporo-parietal and frontal areas were activated with the expert archival paradigm for autobiographical memory recall [13]. Also the right temporoparietal junction (TPJ) and orbitofrontal cortex corresponded to the theory of mind to reason about other's internal state and action rationality evaluation [14]. The TPJ region was found to play important role in complex visual configuration processing for chess experts [15]. In addition, only in the chess experts, interhemispheric correlation such as in the TPJ area was enhanced together with bilateral activation in frontoparietal and occipital regions for accurate chess position visualization [16, 17]. Furthermore, the collateral sulci linked the object position to the spatio-functional environment information stored in memory [18].

And medial prefrontal cortex (MPFC) subserved functional interactions with the amygdala and hippocampus for one's own and social hierarchy learning as well as for the purpose of self-relevant knowledge update [19]. Finally, prolonged electroencephalogram (EEG) signal of N2 and P3 peaks for executive control and selective attention functionalities in chess players were found in response to different chess targets, indicating success pattern matching and memory chunk retrieval in experts [20].

Regarding decision making and global strategy, augmented activation in the inferior parietal cortex (IPC) and lingual gyrus during visual stimulation together with higher striatum and pre-supplementary motor area (SMA) for decision-making facilitation had been reported [21, 22]. Chess masters also exhibited larger inter-striatum-default mode network (DMN) connection, possibly for goal-directed cognitive performance and theory of mind optimization [23]. On the other hand, during chess problem-solving task, DMN connectivity was deactivated but caudate-DMN connectivity was enhanced for possible better high-level cognitive support in chess masters [24]. Enhanced functional connectivity, higher regional homogeneity (ReHo) and fractional amplitude of low frequency fluctuations (fALFF) for local synchronization and neural activity biomarkers reached agreement in several brain regions including posterior fusiform that might benefit from chess expertise [25]. Also large-scale network analysis identified higher clustering coefficient and increased small-worldness properties, possibly due to the increased functional connectivity in the hippocampus/thalamus, basal ganglia and temporo-parietal regions [26]. And better dynamics including higher number of occupancies and longer dwell time in majorities of states were present in chess experts based on dynamic connectome quantification [27].

1.2. Objectives

Imaging evidence of brain cognitive and neuroplasticity changes relating to chess practicing skills and expertise had been reported. The purposes of this chapter are to 1. investigate further brain functional and micro-structural changes in professional chess players compared to controls with available fMRI and DTI data using multiple advanced imaging methods; and 2. correlate the imaging quantifications with phenotypic data in chess players using both voxel-wise and global statistical computation methods and also extend the current knowledge of neuroplasticity and wisdom gain of chess game.

2. Methods

2.1. Participants

Imaging data of 29 chess masters (including usual players) and 29 age- and education level- matched controls were recruited for this project to study brain cognitive function improvements with chess training (Table 1). Imaging and phenotypic data were downloaded after approval from the website managed at the NeuroImaging Tools & Resources Collaboratory (NITRC) database (www.nitrc.org). The multimodal MRI dataset of professional chess players were provided by the Huaxi MR Research Center (HMRRC) at West China Hospital of Sichuan University, as the INDI Prospective Data Sharing Samples hosted by NITRC (http://fcon_1000.projects.nitrc.org/indi/IndiPro.html).

Group	Age (Years)	Gender	Education	Level
Control (N=29)	25.8±1.3	15F, 52%	13.9±0.6 (Y)	4.7±0.2
Chess (N=29)	**Age**	**Gender**	**Education**	**Level**
	28.7±2.0	9F, 31%	13.3±0.5 (Y)	2.3±0.2
	Raven's RPM	**Rate**	**Starting Age**	**Training Time**
	49±1.3	2401.1±28.1	8.6±0.5 (Y)	11.4±2.3 (Y)

* Code for level scale: grand master=1; master=2; play often=3; used to play=4; only know rules =5; don't know rules and never played=6.
In the chess group, 6 grand masters were included with level =1, 11 masters with level =2, 10 players with level =3, 1 with level 4 and 1 with level 5.

Table 1. *Demographic information including age, gender and education levels of two groups as well as phenotypic data including level for amateur controls and professional level for chess group, Raven's progressive matrices (RPM) score, professional rate (in 2009 for this data), starting age of playing and training time of years for chess group.*

No significant differences of age and education levels comparing professional chess group to controls were found, and detailed statistical information of participants of two groups are listed in Table 1. In the chess player group, there were 6 grand masters and 11 masters as well as 10 usual players. There were significant correlations between professional rate and level in chess group (r=-0.670, P<0.001), also between training time and level (r=-0.523, P=0.004) as well as between Raven's progressive matrices (RPM) score and rate (r=0.501, P=0.006).

2.2. Imaging Parameters and Data Processing

MRI experiments were performed using the 3T MRI scanner with standardized imaging protocols. The 3D Magnetization-prepared rapid acquisition gradient-echo (MPRAGE) sequence was run with

TR/TI/TE=1900/900/2.3 ms, flip angle=9°, matrix size=256 x 256 x 176, resolution=1 x 1x 1 mm^3 for reference image used in resting-state (RS)-fMRI activity/connectivity/conductivity maps, as well as for structural voxel-based morphometry (VBM) analysis. For the RS-fMRI data acquired under relaxing condition, a standard gradient-echo EPI sequence (TR/TE=2000/30 msec, flip angle=90°, number of volumes=205, spatial resolution=3.75 x 3.75 x 5 mm^3) was utilized. DTI data was obtained with standard spin-echo EPI sequence (TR/TE=6800/93 msec, flip angle=90°, number of diffusion directions= 42, b-value=1000 s/mm^2, spatial resolution =1.8 x 1.8 x 3.0 mm^3).

The MRI and fMRI images were processed with the in-house developed scripts to derive the voxel-mirrored homotopic correlation (VMHC), VBM, independent component analysis-based dual regression (ICA-DR) remapped components, resting-state functional connectivity (RSFC) and fALFF maps, as described in details from our previous works [19, 20]. Between-group comparisons of quantitative post-processed images were performed with advanced statistical tools using Analysis of Functional NeuroImages (AFNI, http://afni.nimh.nih.gov) package and FMRIB Software Library (FSL, http://www.fmrib.ox.ac.uk/fsl) toolbox. Graph theory based small-worldness systematic analysis was computed to the correlation matrix generated from 116 seeds-based RSFC maps and compared to a degree-matched random network to derive both absolute and relative, local and global efficiency metrics [28, 29].

Novel dynamic functional network correlation (dFNC) connectogram and regional homogeneity (ReHo) map together with typical VMHC, ICA-DR, fALFF, and small-worldness analyses were performed to two data cohorts. The details of data processing were similar to the methods described in our recently published works

[28-31]. For instance, six typical and important functional networks were used for dFNC analysis, including default mode network (DMN), frontoparietal network (FPN), salience network (SN), motor network (MN), visual network (VN) and central executive network (CEN or EN). ReHo map was generated to reflect local synchrony of spontaneous neuronal activities spatially, after preprocessing the fMRI data such as motion correction and low-pass filtering for each voxel of the 4D fMRI data [30, 31].

DTI data were first pre-processed with the Diffusion Toolkit toolbox (http://tractvis.org) to obtain the fractional anisotropy (FA) and three diffusivity metrics such as axial diffusivity (AD), radial diffusivity (RD) and mean diffusivity (MD) values in original B0 diffusion space. For the FA/RD/AD/MD quantification, the FSL tract-based spatial statistics (TBSS) toolbox steps 1–2 (i.e. preprocessing, brain mask extraction with FA>0.1 and normalization) were used for registration of all participants' FA into the FSL 1-mm white matter skeleton template. Statistical comparisons between chess and control groups were performed to the voxel-wise whole brain and 20 tract-based FA/AD/RD/MD data. Correlations between functional and structural/micro-structural imaging data (both voxel-wise and regional/global quantification of statistical Z-values) and phenotypic scales such as professional rate, level and training time were also performed to examine any associations between neural responses and behavior/cognitive metrics [32, 33].

3. Results

VBM results showed significant higher gray matter densities (GMD) in the superior frontal, caudate, cerebellum, occipito-parietal junction, dorsal medial thalamus, supplementary motor area and small orbitofrontal clusters in chess masters compared to controls

(P<0.01, Figure 1A), based on the T1-MPRAGE data. Moreover, higher interhemispheric correlations in the temporal, superior frontal, MPFC, visual, hypothalamus, basal ganglia and cerebellar regions were found in chess masters compared to controls (P<0.05, Figure 1B) with fMRI data. However, lower VMHC in the posterior cingulate, superior parietal and cuneus regions existed in chess masters as well.

Using ICA-DR algorithm, higher inter- and intra- network connectivities of visual, thalamocortical including temporal and sensory regions, DMN-MPFC, salience network-superior temporal, and superior frontal regions were present in the chess players compared to controls (P<0.05, Figure 2). Lower inter-network connectivities of thalamo-occipital/frontal, DMN-visual, fronto-motor and cerebellum regions existed on the other hand, for possible rerouting, deactivation and inhibition function. Also based on relatively new dFNC analysis, higher dynamic correlations between SN-CEN, SN-DMN, FPN-MN and VN-DMN of fMRI correlation matrices data existed in chess masters compared to controls at representative state S3, with relatively lower inter- MN-VN connection (Figure 3). Similar network connectivity patterns were found in both controls and chess masters in another representative state S4, with slightly higher SN-MN and FPN-VN but lower FPN-SN inter-network connectivities in chess master compared to controls. Evenly distributed cluster occurrences in all six states were present in controls (Figure 4 A1, 16-18%); while evenly distributed in five states (Figure 4 B1, 17-22%) but quite lower in one state (3%) were found in chess masters. Relatively longer mean dwell time in majorities of states was observed in chess masters compared to controls, with higher frequency found in most states as well (Figure 4; B1 and B2 respectively).

Higher global mean Z-values of ReHo, VMHC, fALFF and sub-bands S4/S5 were observed in chess master group compared to control group. Significantly higher global mean Z-values (P<0.01) of ReHo and fALFF sub-band S5 in chess masters compared to controls were displayed in Figure 5A, and strong correlations between global Z-values of ReHo and fALFF in chess masters including all fALFF sub-bands (S4 and S5) and conventional band (all r>0.48, P<0.009) were demonstrated in Figure 5B. No other significant voxel-wise functional homogeneity, activity or connectivity differences between chess and control groups were found with P>0.05. In addition, graph-theory based small-worldness analysis of the fMRI correlational data presented higher absolute local but lower relative global efficiencies in chess masters compared to control group (Figure 6A), together with slightly lower small-worldness weighting factor in chess master group (Figure 6B). Significantly higher absolute local efficiency at all sparsity levels in chess masters compared to controls were observed (P=0.02).

Applying statistical correlational analysis to the whole brain voxel-wise imaging data, strong associations between phenotypic scores (mainly for chess master players) and fALFF values (marker for the neuronal activity) were observed. For instance, positive correlations between starting age and fALFF values in the temporo-occipital, subcortical putamen as well as cingulate areas, between professional rate scale and fALFF in temporal/cerebellar cluster, between professional level and temporal fALFF, between Raven's RPM score and fALFF values in the posterior cingulate/precuneus and MFPC, training time and left superior parietal regions were observed (Figure 7A, P<0.05). Also negative correlations between rate scale and occipital fALFF, between Raven's RPM score and sensorimotor fALFF, between training time and temporal fALFF existed. For the VBM results, chess master level correlated with gray matter density (GMD) in the dorsolateral and medial prefrontal regions but linked to GMD of sensorimotor areas in control group and even negative association in the subcortical caudate region (Figure 7B, P<0.05). Positive correlation between GMD in occipital /temporal regions and Raven's RPM score in chess group was found. Furthermore, negative correlations between rate scale and gray matter densities in the dorsolateral prefrontal cortex, between Raven's score and basal ganglia gray matter, between training time and gray matter densities in the frontotemporal and motor areas were observed as well.

Figure 8 demonstrated the phenotypic associations with fMRI ReHo and VMHC quantification (left and right panel respectively), and mainly for chess master group with P<0.05. For instance, significant positive correlations between ReHo and chess professional level were exhibited in the medial/superior frontal region, and similarly for professional rate score in the small cerebellum. Starting age also correlated negatively to the regional homogeneity (ReHo) in the insular, superior temporal and premotor/motor areas, but positively to the ReHo values in the supplementary motor area, subcortical caudate and occipital cortex. Strong associations with negative correlations between Raven's RPM score and ReHo in the frontal/motor areas/small temporal clusters, between training time and superior frontal ReHo were also found (Figure 8A). For the VMHC, strong positive correlations between professional level and frontal/occipital interhemispheric correlation were identified in master group, but only frontal conductivity correlated with level scale in the control group. As expected, starting age was negatively related to VMHC in the regions of insular and superior temporal cortex (salience network), cuneus, sensorimotor and language Wernicke's and Broca's areas in chess group (Figure 8B). Moreover, Raven's RPM score correlated positively with superior temporal VMHC, and training time was linked to VMHC in large areas of frontotemporal and thalamic regions.

Based on TBSS analysis, significantly higher FA (corrected P<0.05) values in several brain tracts were found in chess masters compared to controls, including arcuate fasciculus, cingulum, inferior longitudinal, inferior fronto-occipital fasciculus, corpus callosum and cortico-spinal tracts (Figure 9). Significant correlations between quantitative DTI metrics including 20 tracts-specific mean FA/AD/RD/MD values and phenotypic scores in controls and mostly chess masters are illustrated in Figure 10. For instance, significant links between bilateral inferior longitudinal fasciculus diffusivity (AD/RD/MD) and training time/professional level ($|r|≥0.48$, $P≤0.008$) in chess group; as well as between bilateral SLF diffusivity and training time/ professional level ($|r|≥0.48$, $P≤0.008$) were observed. In addition, the right cingulum FA/MD values were associated with training time in chess group (($|r|≥0.51$, $P≤0.004$). However, FA of right cingulum connecting the hippocampus correlated positively with professional level ($r=0.50$, $P=0.006$) in controls, but radial diffusivity (RD) correlated negatively with level ($r=-0.51$, $P=0.005$; and similar to chess group). The quantitative significant correlations ($P<0.01$) are also listed in Table 2.

Tract Name	Phenotypic Data	DTI	r	P
Cingulum R	training time	FA	0.5420	0.0024
		RD	-0.5140	0.0043
Inferior longitudinal fasciculus L	professional level	MD	0.4830	0.0080
	training time	RD	-0.5480	0.0021
		MD	-0.5420	0.0024
Inferior longitudinal fasciculus R	training time	RD	-0.4850	0.0076
		AD	-0.5720	0.0012
		MD	-0.5490	0.0021
Superior longitudinal fasciculus (temporal part) L	professional level	AD	0.4840	0.0079
	training time	MD	-0.4830	0.0079
Superior longitudinal fasciculus (temporal part) R	professional level	MD	0.4970	0.0061
	training time		-0.5210	0.0037
Forceps major	*professional level in controls*	*FA*	*0.4970*	*0.0061*
Cingulum (hippocampus) R		*RD*	*-0.5100*	*0.0047*

Table 2. *Significant correlations (P<0.01) between phenotypic data and DTI tracts with four metrics of DTI (FA, MD, AD and RD) and 20 tracts in chess group (first 12 rows) and control group (last two rows). L=left, R=right.*

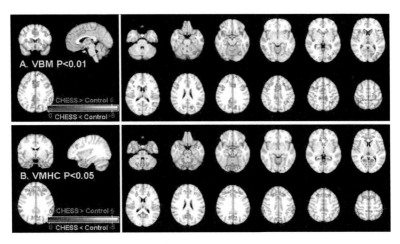

Figure 1. *A: VBM results showed significant higher gray matter densities in the superior frontal, caudate, cerebellum, occipito-parietal junction, dorsal medial thalamus, supplementary motor area and small orbitofrontal clusters in chess masters compared to controls (P<0.01). B: Higher interhemispheric correlations in the temporal, MPFC, superior frontal, visual hypothalamus, basal ganglia and cerebellar regions were found in chess masters compared to controls (P<0.05). On the other hand, lower VMHC in the posterior cingulate, superior parietal and cuneus regions existed as well.*

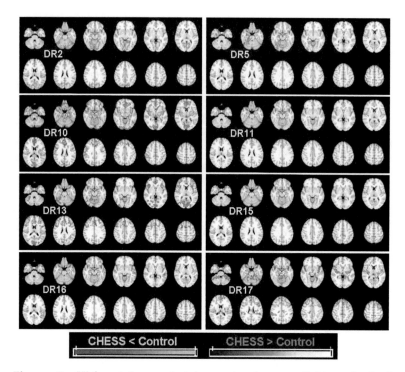

Figure 2. *Higher inter- and intra- network connectivities of visual, thalamocortical including temporal and sensory regions, DMN-medial prefrontal, salience network-superior temporal, and superior frontal areas were present in the chess players compared to controls (P<0.05). Lower inter-network connectivities of thalamo-occipital/frontal, DMN-visual, fronto-motor and cerebellum regions also existed.*

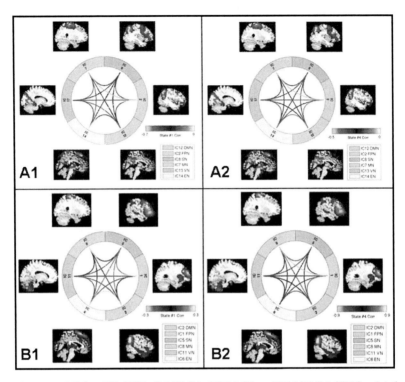

Figure 3. *Higher SN-CEN, SN-DMN, FPN-MN and VN-DMN dFNC existed in chess masters compared to controls at state S3 (B1 vs. A1), with relatively lower inter- MN-VN connectivity. Similar network connectivity patterns were found in both controls and chess masters at state S4 (A2 and B2), with slightly higher SN-MN and FPN-VN but lower FPN-SN dynamic connections in chess masters.*

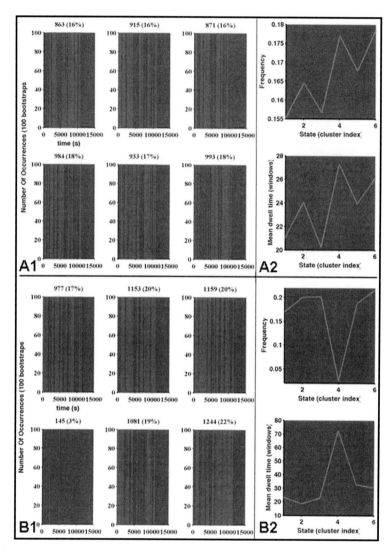

Figure 4. *Evenly distributed cluster occurrences in all six states were present in controls (A1, 16-18%); while evenly distributed in five states (B1, 17-22%) but quite lower in one state (3%) in chess masters. Relatively longer mean dwell time in majorities of states in chess masters compared to controls, with higher frequency in most states (B1 and B2 respectively).*

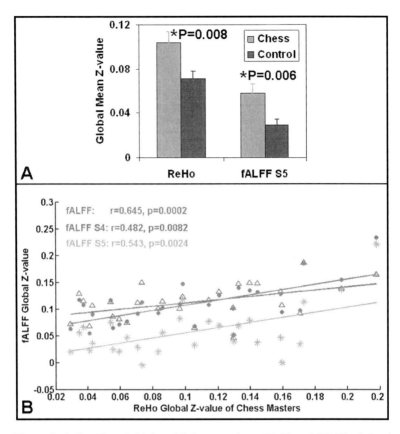

Figure 5. *A: Significantly higher global mean values of ReHo and fALFF sub-band S5 in chess masters compared to controls (P=0.008 and P=0.006 respectively). B: Strong correlations between global Z-values of ReHo and fALFF in chess masters including all fALFF sub-bands (S4 and S5) and conventional band (r>0.48, P<0.009).*

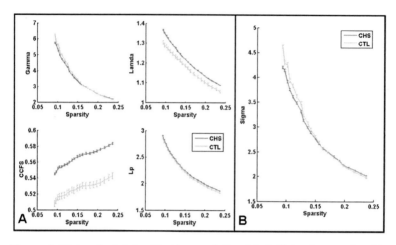

Figure 6. *Higher absolute local but lower relative global efficiencies were found in chess masters compared to control group (A), together with slightly lower small-worldness weighting factor in chess master group (B).*

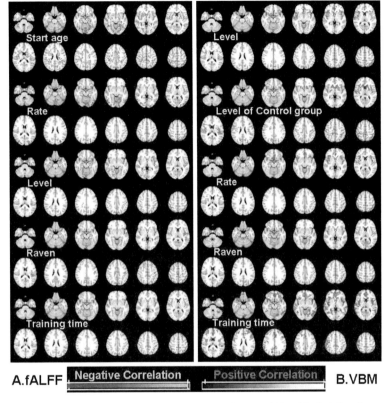

A.fALFF   Negative Correlation   Positive Correlation   B.VBM

Figure 7. *Correlation maps of fALFF (A) and VBM (B) with P<0.05. Strong correlations between start age and fALFF values in the temporo-occipital, subcortical putamen and cingulate areas were observed. Positive correlations between rate scale and fALFF of small areas in the cerebellum/temporal clusters; level and fALFF in the temporal together with Raven's RPM score and posterior cingulate/ precuneus, medial frontal fALFF, training time and left superior parietal regions were observed. Negative correlations existed between rate scale and occipital fALFF, between Raven's RPM score and sensorimotor fALFF, between training time and temporal fALFF as well. For VBM, master level correlated with gray matter density in the dorsolateral and medial prefrontal regions, while with sensorimotor areas in control group (and even negative in the caudate region). Negative correlations between rate scale and gray matter densities in the dorsolateral prefrontal cortex, between Raven's score and basal ganglia gray matter, between training time and gray matter densities in the frontotemporal and* *motor areas but positive association between occipital VBM and Raven's score were observed as well.*

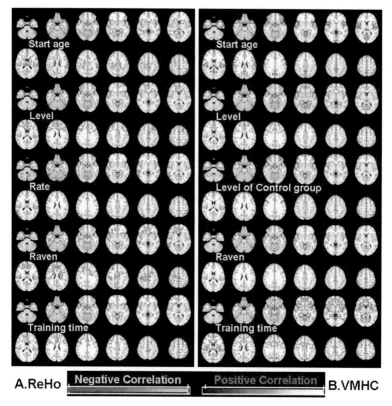

Figure 8. *Correlation maps of ReHo (A) and VMHC (B) for chess master group with P<0.05. For instance, significant positive correlations between ReHo and chess professional level were exhibited in the medial/superior frontal regions, and similarly for professional rate score in the small cerebellum. Starting age also correlated negatively with insular/superior temporal/premotor ReHo values but positively in the supplementary motor area, subcortical caudate and occipital cortex. Strong associations with negative correlations between Raven's RPM score and ReHo in the frontal/motor areas and small temporal clusters, between training time and superior frontal ReHo were also found. For the VMHC, strong positive correlations between professional level and frontal/occipital interhemispheric correlation in master group, but only frontal conductivity with level in the control*

group were identified. As expected, starting age was negatively related to VMHC in the regions of insular and superior temporal cortex (salience network), cuneus and sensorimotor and language Wernicke's and Broca's areas. Raven's RPM score correlated positively with superior temporal VMHC, and training time was linked to large areas of frontotemporal and thalamic regions.

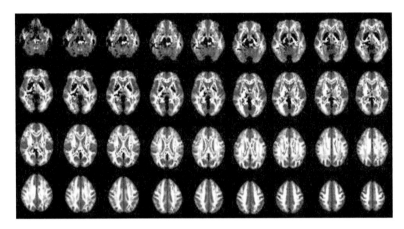

Figure 9. *Higher FA in several brain tracts were found in chess masters compared to controls, including arcuate fasciculus, cingulum, inferior longitudinal fasciculus, inferior fronto-occipital fasciculus, corpus callosum and cortico-spinal tracts (corrected P<0.05).*

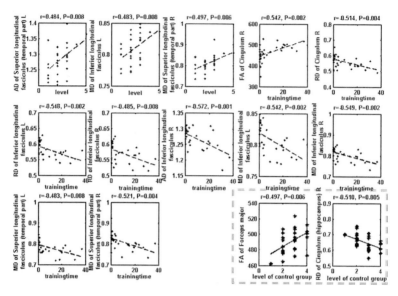

Figure 10. *Significant correlations between DTI metrics and phenotypic data in chess masters mainly (P<0.01), and for controls (red dashed box of the right bottom panel). Expected correlations in chess group but reversal directions in control groups were found, possibly reflecting the sub-optimal memory and motor pathways in controls.*

4. Discussion

4.1. Summary of Results

In this project, we found consistent gray matter densities and interhemispheric correlation changes in chess players compared to controls, including both higher in the superior frontal, MPFC and visual/cerebellum regions. The VMHC identified extra hypo-connectivity in the parietal and cuneus regions but hyper-conductivity in the temporal and subcortical basal ganglia and hypothalamus, while VBM localized further higher gray matter densities in the orbitofrontal, caudate, cuneus and supplementary motor areas in the chess group. These primarily increased gray matter densities and conductivity in critical brain regions indicated expected improvement of high-level cognitive functions including decision planning and making (supplementary motor and superior frontal areas), memory and attention (posterior temporal and orbitofrontal cortices), visuospatial ability (occipital lobe), reasoning and movement coordination (MPFC, subcortical and cerebellum) in chess masters.

In line with the structural/conductivity changes, increased intra- and inter-network connectivities of several crucial brain networks were illustrated with the ICA-DR algorithm, including visual network (VN), central executive network (CEN), thalamocortical circuits such as motor network (MN), default mode network (DMN)-medial frontal region, frontoparietal network (FPN) as well as the salience network (SN) in the chess players compared to controls. The relatively new dFNC built on these six networks also confirmed higher dynamic correlations between SN-CEN, SN-DMN, FPN-MN and VN-DMN in chess masters compared to controls. The overall dwell time and occurrence number were longer in majorities of states (5 out of 6) in chess group compared to controls, utilizing the strategy of setting one dip state with lowest occurrence number/dwell time and maintaining higher dynamics for other five states. Furthermore, significantly higher global regional homogeneity (ReHo, local synchrony) and neural activity (fALFF) were found in chess group compared to controls, with strong correlations between these two metrics. And much higher absolute local efficiency was noticed in chess group with close small-worldness factor and global efficiency between two groups. Higher global neural activity/regional synchrony in chess group with increased local efficiency indicated better and fast neuronal source allocation and utilization. The expected higher inter-network connectivity of DMN, CEN, SN, VN and FPN with longer mean dynamic state time and more occurrence number confirmed both static and dynamic network regulation improvements in chess group compared to controls, particularly in the domains of decision making, attention and memory, vision and wisdom.

Multiple couplings between brain activity/connectivity and phenotypic data had been revealed in chess group, and were in agreement with the functionalities of these regions. For instance, associations were observed between Raven's RPM score and neural activity in the superior frontal and posterior cingulate region as well as between Raven's RPM score and gray matter density in the temporal and occipital clusters. Professional rate correlated positively with cerebellar regional synchrony, while starting age was negatively related to the interhemispheric conductivity in the salience network and temporal/cuneus region. Some other correlations existed such as positive correlations between levels and frontal VMHC, between start age and subcortical ReHo/fALFF, possibly due to neuroprotective and compensatory mechanisms. Finally, consistent whole voxel-wise and regional tract-specific DTI FA increments were present in chess group, including the arcuate fasciculus, inferior longitudinal and inferior fronto-occipital fascicle, corpus callosum and cortico-spinal tracts. Tight links between DTI FA/diffusivity (AD/RD/MD) metrics and phenotypic data were discovered, including between bilateral inferior longitudinal fasciculus/cingulum diffusivity/FA and training time/professional level in chess group. The DTI microstructural findings confirmed improvement of brain memory, language and communication function, decision making and processing speed due to practice and professional training.

4.2. Comparison with Previous Findings

Recent studies had also showed superior abilities in chess masters compared to non-chess players with better auditory memory function and higher planning performance scores [34, 35]. A few underlying mechanism for these advantages were also evaluated including pattern recognition training as part of the chess expertise, together with effective working memory retrieval and neuroplasticity gain between short and long term memory encoding processes [36]. The memory chunk hypothesis, especially in chess grand masters that could achieve magic and fast retrieval of large quantities of board and piece templates stored in short and long-term brain memory regions, might help explain the proficient chess expert memory structure [37, 38]. The expertise theory was also in agreement with the findings and indicated successful operation of very large chunk (such as 50,000 templates) in chess maters and recall of position-specific pattern [39, 40]. The beneficial influences of chess on brain, behavior and possible therapeutic tool had further been discussed, especially with the evidence of brain alterations for better cognitive performance and accurate decision-making process [41]. For instance, associated brain changes in chess experts were manifested as cerebral blood flow reorganization due to the encouragement of utilizing or transferring partial long-term memory as working memory, as well as joint regional activation in the superior frontoparietal and precuneal clusters corresponding to both small- and large-scale spatial capability acceleration [42-43]. Similar white matter changes as observed in our results and a recent study had also confirmed training effects on microstructural integrity improvements, particularly in tracts of superior longitudinal fasciculus, inferior longitudinal fasciculus and cingulum for memory and executive functions as well as visual/cognitive abilities [44].

For the other games-related brain changes, increased FA in the frontal, cingulum and striatal-thalamic areas were identified and linked to attentional control, working memory, executive regulation and problem solving in Baduk GO game experts compared to controls [45]. In internet gaming disorders (IGD), thalamocortical communication was abnormally increased and the hyper-connectivity between midline nucleus/postcentral gyrus correlated with less inhibition scores [46]. Also it had further been confirmed that several cortical networks were disrupted, such as FPN and temporal/dorsal-limbic networks that were positively related to IGD scores as well as game craving score [47, 48]. The anterior cingulate cortex (ACC) activation generated feedback-related negativity, functioning as possible loss cue compared to win sign as well as the alert signal to urge for preparation of future events [49]. Some social-economical and neuropsychological related issues including long-term morality and reward topics were discussed recently; for instance, social status including social norms during fairness perception correlated with the connectivity between right anterior insular (rAI) and ACC while rAI sent regulatory signal to ACC and amygdala at unintentional situation [50, 51]. The positive correlation between ventral striatum activation and fairness was reduced at losing condition, but negative association between dorsolateral prefrontal activation and fairness was enhanced [52]. The context-dependent processing of social and metalizing processes involved insula and dorsolateral prefrontal cortex (DLPFC) primarily, with more activations observed under high pressures [53]. These two regions also affected both self-interest and other-need concerns, responsible for evaluating the benefactor's altruistic decisions under risks and ambiguity [54, 55].

4.3. Conclusion

In this study, we had reported brain associated structural and functional network optimization in chess players compared to controls. Especially, higher gray matter density and interhemispheric correlation in the superior frontal region, medial prefrontal cortex, supplementary motor area, temporal lobe and cerebellum, orbitofrontal and occipital areas that were associated with better cognitive functions in the memory and attention, decision making and visuospatial ability, executive control and movement coordination. Increased dynamic correlations of typical brain networks such as VN, CEN, MN and DMN/CEN together with longer dwell time/occupancy/frequency for optimal strategy in chess players had also been confirmed. Moreover, global neural activity and regional synchrony signals were enhanced in chess professionals compared to controls, together with the higher absolute local efficiency for faster local neural source utilization. Micro-structural integrity was improved in several tracts including cingulum, corpus callosum, inferior and superior longitudinal fascicle in chess group. And these neural activity, functional/ microstructural connectivity and conductivity alterations were strongly related to the phenotypic data such as training time and professional level. Our comprehensive results complemented previous findings, validating the multi-level gains including static and dynamic, local and global, structural and functional perspectives for essential brain and behavior competence in chess training, practice and expertise.

References

[1] Li K, Jiang J, Qiu L, Yang X, Huang X, Lui S, Gong Q. A multimodal MRI dataset of professional chess players. Sci Data. 2015 Sep 1;2:150044. doi: 10.1038/sdata.2015.44. PMID: 26346238; PMCID: PMC4556927.

[2] Mayeli M, Rahmani F, Aarabi MH. Comprehensive Investigation of White Matter Tracts in Professional Chess Players and Relation to Expertise: Region of Interest and DMRI Connectometry. Front Neurosci. 2018 May 3;12:288. doi: 10.3389/fnins.2018.00288. PMID: 29773973; PMCID: PMC5943529.

[3] Hänggi J, Brütsch K, Siegel AM, Jäncke L. The architecture of the chess player's brain. Neuropsychologia. 2014 Sep;62:152-62. doi: 10.1016/j.neuropsychologia.2014.07.019. Epub 2014 Jul 24. PMID: 25065494.

[4] Grabner RH, Neubauer AC, Stern E. Superior performance and neural efficiency: the impact of intelligence and expertise. Brain Res Bull. 2006 Apr 28;69(4):422-39. doi: 10.1016/j.brainresbull.2006.02.009. Epub 2006 Mar 3. PMID: 16624674.

[5] Gong Y, Ericsson KA, Moxley JH. Recall of briefly presented chess positions and its relation to chess skill. PLoS One. 2015 Mar 16;10(3):e0118756. doi: 10.1371/journal.pone.0118756. PMID: 25774693; PMCID: PMC4361603.

[6] RaviPrakash H, Anwar SM, Biassou NM, Bagci U. Morphometric and Functional Brain Connectivity Differentiates Chess Masters From Amateur Players. Front Neurosci. 2021 Feb 19;15:629478. doi: 10.3389/fnins.2021.629478. PMID: 33679310; PMCID: PMC7933502.

[7] Ouellette DJ, Hsu DL, Stefancin P, Duong TQ. Cortical thickness and functional connectivity changes in Chinese chess experts. PLoS One. 2020 Oct 7;15(10):e0239822. doi: 10.1371/journal.pone.0239822. PMID: 33027295; PMCID: PMC7540889.

[8] Bilalić M, Turella L, Campitelli G, Erb M, Grodd W. Expertise modulates the neural basis of context dependent recognition of objects and their relations. Hum Brain Mapp. 2012 Nov;33(11):2728-40. doi: 10.1002/hbm.21396. Epub 2011 Oct 13. PMID: 21998070; PMCID: PMC6870017.

[9] Bilalić M, Langner R, Ulrich R, Grodd W. Many faces of expertise: fusiform face area in chess experts and novices. J Neurosci. 2011 Jul

13;31(28):10206-14. doi: 10.1523/JNEUROSCI.5727-10.2011. PMID: 21752997; PMCID: PMC6623046.

[10] Bilalić M, Langner R, Erb M, Grodd W. Mechanisms and neural basis of object and pattern recognition: a study with chess experts. J Exp Psychol Gen. 2010 Nov;139(4):728-42. doi: 10.1037/a0020756. PMID: 21038986.

[11] Campitelli G, Gobet F, Head K, Buckley M, Parker A. Brain localization of memory chunks in chessplayers. Int J Neurosci. 2007 Dec;117(12):1641-59. doi: 10.1080/00207450601041955. PMID: 17987468.

[12] Campitelli G, Gobet F, Parker A. Structure and stimulus familiarity: a study of memory in chess-players with functional magnetic resonance imaging. Span J Psychol. 2005 Nov;8(2):238-45. doi: 10.1017/s1138741600005126. PMID: 16255391.

[13] Campitelli G, Parker A, Head K, Gobet F. Left lateralization in autobiographical memory: an fMRI study using the expert archival paradigm. Int J Neurosci. 2008 Feb;118(2):191-209. doi: 10.1080/00207450701668053. PMID: 18205077.

[14] Powell JL, Grossi D, Corcoran R, Gobet F, García-Fiñana M. The neural correlates of theory of mind and their role during empathy and the game of chess: A functional magnetic resonance imaging study. Neuroscience. 2017 Jul 4;355:149-160. doi: 10.1016/j.neuroscience.2017.04.042. Epub 2017 May 8. PMID: 28495332.

[15] Rennig J, Bilalić M, Huberle E, Karnath HO, Himmelbach M. The temporo-parietal junction contributes to global gestalt perception-evidence from studies in chess experts. Front Hum Neurosci. 2013 Aug 28;7:513. doi: 10.3389/fnhum.2013.00513. PMID: 24009574; PMCID: PMC3755212.

[16] Bilalić M, Kiesel A, Pohl C, Erb M, Grodd W. It takes two-skilled recognition of objects engages lateral areas in both hemispheres. PLoS One. 2011 Jan 24;6(1):e16202. doi: 10.1371/journal.pone.0016202. PMID: 21283683; PMCID: PMC3025982.

[17] Atherton M, Zhuang J, Bart WM, Hu X, He S. A functional MRI study of high-level cognition. I. The game of chess. Brain Res Cogn Brain Res. 2003 Mar;16(1):26-31. doi: 10.1016/s0926-6410(02)00207-0. PMID: 12589885.

[18] Langner R, Eickhoff SB, Bilalić M. A network view on brain regions involved in experts' object and pattern recognition: Implications for the neural mechanisms of skilled visual perception. Brain Cogn. 2019 Apr;131:74-86. doi: 10.1016/j.bandc.2018.09.007. Epub 2018 Oct 2. PMID: 30290974; PMCID: PMC6421106.

[19] Kumaran D, Banino A, Blundell C, Hassabis D, Dayan P. Computations Underlying Social Hierarchy Learning: Distinct Neural Mechanisms for Updating and Representing Self-Relevant Information. Neuron. 2016 Dec 7;92(5):1135-1147. doi: 10.1016/j.neuron.2016.10.052. PMID: 27930904; PMCID: PMC5158095.

[20] Wright MJ, Gobet F, Chassy P, Ramchandani PN. ERP to chess stimuli reveal expert-novice differences in the amplitudes of N2 and P3 components. Psychophysiology. 2013 Oct;50(10):1023-33. doi: 10.1111/psyp.12084. Epub 2013 Jul 10. PMID: 23837745.

[21] Neumann N, Lotze M, Eickhoff SB. Cognitive Expertise: An ALE Meta-Analysis. Hum Brain Mapp. 2016 Jan;37(1):262-72. doi: 10.1002/hbm.23028. Epub 2015 Oct 14. PMID: 26467981; PMCID: PMC6867472.

[22] Forstmann BU, Dutilh G, Brown S, Neumann J, von Cramon DY, Ridderinkhof KR, Wagenmakers EJ. Striatum and pre-SMA facilitate decision-making under time pressure. Proc Natl Acad Sci U S A. 2008 Nov 11;105(45):17538-42. doi: 10.1073/pnas.0805903105. Epub 2008 Nov 3. PMID: 18981414; PMCID: PMC2582260.

[23] Duan X, He S, Liao W, Liang D, Qiu L, Wei L, Li Y, Liu C, Gong Q, Chen H. Reduced caudate volume and enhanced striatal-DMN integration in chess experts. Neuroimage. 2012 Apr 2;60(2):1280-6. doi: 10.1016/j.neuroimage.2012.01.047. Epub 2012 Jan 14. PMID: 22270350.

[24] Duan X, Liao W, Liang D, Qiu L, Gao Q, Liu C, Gong Q, Chen H. Large-scale brain networks in board game experts: insights from a domain-related task and task-free resting state. PLoS One. 2012;7(3):e32532. doi: 10.1371/journal.pone.0032532. Epub 2012 Mar 12. PMID: 22427852; PMCID: PMC3299676.

[25] Song L, Peng Q, Liu S, Wang J. Changed hub and functional connectivity patterns of the posterior fusiform gyrus in chess experts. Brain Imaging Behav. 2020 Jun;14(3):797-805. doi: 10.1007/s11682-018-0020-0. PMID: 30612341.

[26] Duan X, Long Z, Chen H, Liang D, Qiu L, Huang X, Liu TC, Gong Q. Functional organization of intrinsic connectivity networks in Chinese-chess experts. Brain Res. 2014 Apr 16;1558:33-43. doi: 10.1016/ j.brainres.2014.02.033. Epub 2014 Feb 22. PMID: 24565926.

[27] Premi E, Gazzina S, Diano M, Girelli A, Calhoun VD, Iraji A, Gong Q, Li K, Cauda F, Gasparotti R, Padovani A, Borroni B, Magoni M. Enhanced dynamic functional connectivity (whole-brain chronnectome) in chess experts. Sci Rep. 2020 Apr 27;10(1):7051. doi: 10.1038/s41598-020-63984-8. PMID: 32341444; PMCID: PMC7184623.

[28] Zhou Y. *Functional Neuroimaging with Multiple Modalities: Principle, Device and Applications.* Nova Science Publishers. 2016.

[29] Zhou Y. *Imaging and Multiomic Biomarker Applications: Advances in Early Alzheimer's Disease.* Nova Science Publishers. 2020.

[30] Zhou Y. *Typical Imaging in Atypical Parkinson's, Schizophrenia, Epilepsy and Asymptomatic Alzheimer's Disease.* Nova Science Publishers. 2021.

[31] Zhou Y. *Functional Neuroimaging Methods and Frontiers.* Nova Science Publishers. 2018.

[32] Zhou Y. *Joint Imaging Applications in General Neurodegenerative Disease: Parkinson's, Frontotemporal, Vascular Dementia and Autism.* Nova Science Publishers. 2021.

[33] Zhou Y. Multiparametric Imaging in Neurodegenerative Disease. Nova Science Publishers. 2019.

[34] Fattahi F, Geshani A, Jafari Z, Jalaie S, Salman Mahini M. Auditory memory function in expert chess players. Med J Islam Repub Iran. 2015 Oct 6;29:275. PMID: 26793666; PMCID: PMC4715404.

[35] Unterrainer JM, Kaller CP, Halsband U, Rahm B. Planning abilities and chess: a comparison of chess and non-chess players on the Tower of London task. Br J Psychol. 2006 Aug;97(Pt 3):299-311. doi: 10.1348/000712605X71407. PMID: 16848944.

[36] Schultetus RS, Charness N. Recall or evaluation of chess positions revisited: the relationship between memory and evaluation in chess skill. Am J Psychol. 1999 Winter;112(4):555-69. PMID: 10696266.

[37] Gobet F, Simon HA. Templates in chess memory: a mechanism for recalling several boards. Cogn Psychol. 1996 Aug;31(1):1-40. doi: 10.1006/cogp.1996.0011. PMID: 8812020.

[38] Gobet F, Simon HA. Expert chess memory: revisiting the chunking hypothesis. Memory. 1998 May;6(3):225-55. doi: 10.1080/741942359. PMID: 9709441.

[39] Gobet F, Clarkson G. Chunks in expert memory: evidence for the magical number four ... or is it two? Memory. 2004 Nov;12(6):732-47. doi: 10.1080/09658210344000530. PMID: 15724362.

[40] Gobet F, Simon HA. Recall of random and distorted chess positions: implications for the theory of expertise. Mem Cognit. 1996 Jul;24(4):493-503. doi: 10.3758/bf03200937. PMID: 8757497.

[41] Franklin GL, Pereira BNGV, Lima NSC, Germiniani FMB, Camargo CHF, Caramelli P, Teive HAG. Neurology, psychiatry and the chess game: a narrative review. Arq Neuropsiquiatr. 2020 Mar;78(3):169-175. doi: 10.1590/0004-282x20190187. Epub 2020 Apr 27. PMID: 32348415.

[42] Guida A, Gobet F, Tardieu H, Nicolas S. How chunks, long-term working memory and templates offer a cognitive explanation for neuroimaging data on expertise acquisition: a two-stage framework. Brain Cogn. 2012 Aug;79(3):221-44. doi: 10.1016/j.bandc.2012.01.010. Epub 2012

[43] Li Y, Kong F, Ji M, Luo Y, Lan J, You X. Shared and Distinct Neural Bases of Large- and Small-Scale Spatial Ability: A Coordinate-Based Activation Likelihood Estimation Meta-Analysis. Front Neurosci. 2019 Jan 10;12:1021. doi: 10.3389/fnins.2018.01021. PMID: 30686987; PMCID: PMC6335367.

[44] Zhou S, Jin L, He J, Zeng Q, Wu Y, Cao Z, Feng Y. Distributed performance of white matter properties in chess players: A DWI study using automated fiber quantification. Brain Res. 2018 Dec 1;1700:9-18. doi: 10.1016/j.brainres.2018.07.003. Epub 2018 Jul 7. PMID: 29990490.

[45] Lee B, Park JY, Jung WH, Kim HS, Oh JS, Choi CH, Jang JH, Kang DH, Kwon JS. White matter neuroplastic changes in long-term trained players of the game of "Baduk" (GO): a voxel-based diffusion-tensor imaging study. Neuroimage. 2010 Aug 1;52(1):9-19. doi: 10.1016/j.neuroimage.2010.04.014. Epub 2010 Apr 13. PMID: 20394826.

[46] Zhou W, Zheng H, Wang M, Zheng Y, Chen S, Wang MJ, Dong GH. The imbalance between goal-directed and habitual systems in internet gaming disorder: Results from the disturbed thalamocortical

communications. J Psychiatr Res. 2021 Feb;134:121-128. doi: 10.1016/j.jpsychires.2020.12.058. Epub 2020 Dec 22. PMID: 33383495.

[47] Ma SS, Worhunsky PD, Xu JS, Yip SW, Zhou N, Zhang JT, Liu L, Wang LJ, Liu B, Yao YW, Zhang S, Fang XY. Alterations in functional networks during cue-reactivity in Internet gaming disorder. J Behav Addict. 2019 Jun 1;8(2):277-287. doi: 10.1556/2006.8.2019.25. Epub 2019 May 31. PMID: 31146550; PMCID: PMC7044545.

[48] Wang Y, Yang LQ, Li S, Zhou Y. Game Theory Paradigm: A New Tool for Investigating Social Dysfunction in Major Depressive Disorders. Front Psychiatry. 2015 Sep 15;6:128. doi: 10.3389/fpsyt.2015.00128. PMID: 26441689; PMCID: PMC4569817

[49] Yu R, Zhou X. Brain potentials associated with outcome expectation and outcome evaluation. Neuroreport. 2006 Oct 23;17(15):1649-53. doi: 10.1097/01.wnr.0000236866. 39328.1d. PMID: 17001286.

[50] Hu J, Blue PR, Yu H, Gong X, Xiang Y, Jiang C, Zhou X. Social status modulates the neural response to unfairness. Soc Cogn Affect Neurosci. 2016 Jan;11(1):1-10. doi: 10.1093/scan/nsv086. Epub 2015 Jul 2. PMID: 26141925; PMCID: PMC4692311.

[51] Yu H, Li J, Zhou X. Neural substrates of intention--consequence integration and its impact on reactive punishment in interpersonal transgression. J Neurosci. 2015 Mar 25;35(12): 4917-25. doi: 10.1523/JNEUROSCI.3536-14.2015. Erratum in: J Neurosci. 2015 Jun 10;35(23):8970. PMID: 25810522; PMCID: PMC6705376.

[52] Wu Y, Yu H, Shen B, Yu R, Zhou Z, Zhang G, Jiang Y, Zhou X. Neural basis of increased costly norm enforcement under adversity. Soc Cogn Affect Neurosci. 2014 Dec;9(12):1862-71. doi: 10.1093/ scan/nst187. Epub 2014 Jan 5. PMID: 24396005; PMCID: PMC4249466.

[53] Gao X, Yu H, Sáez I, Blue PR, Zhu L, Hsu M, Zhou X. Distinguishing neural correlates of context-dependent advantageous- and disadvantageous-inequity aversion. Proc Natl Acad Sci U S A. 2018 Aug 14;115(33):E7680-E7689. doi: 10.1073/pnas.1802523115. Epub 2018 Jul 30. PMID: 30061413; PMCID: PMC6099874. [54

[54] Xiong W, Gao X, He Z, Yu H, Liu H, Zhou X. Affective evaluation of others' altruistic decisions under risk and ambiguity. Neuroimage. 2020 Sep;218:116996. doi: 10.1016/j.neuroimage.2020.116996. Epub 2020 May 26. PMID: 32470571.

[55] Hu J, Li Y, Yin Y, Blue PR, Yu H, Zhou X. How do self-interest and other-need interact in the brain to determine altruistic behavior? Neuroimage. 2017 Aug 15;157:598-611. doi: 10.1016/j.neuroimage. 2017.06.040. Epub 2017 Jun 20. PMID: 28645841.

Chapter 2
Brain Activation of Music, Counting and Memory Tasks

Abstract

In this work, we had performed all six conditional VMHC comparisons, including each of three task conditions vs. resting state, as well as between two-task comparisons. Similar brain patterns of lower VMHC in the visual, temporal and somatosensory, motor areas under music/counting/memory tasks compared to resting state were observed. Between-comparisons for each two of three tasks further demonstrated the distinct regional allocation of neural resources. For instance, medial prefrontal, anterior cingulate, insular, superior temporal, occipital, thalamus, cerebellum and motor/supplementary motor areas related to music singing, with more differences comparing music to counting than memory tasks. The counting task also revealed more orbitofrontal interhemispheric correlation in addition to specific intra-parietal sulcus (IPS) and superior frontal gyrus (SFG) conductivity compared to music/memory. While clusters in the medial temporal lobe including hippocampus and parahippocampus, posterior cingulate, precuneus, dorsolateral prefrontal cortex (DLPFC) and superior parietal lobe maintained higher VMHC during episodic memory recall processing than music and counting tasks.

Functional connectivity based ICA-DR algorithm identified enhanced network connectivities of intra- DMN, FPN and SN during music singing condition compared to counting and memory recall tasks. On the other hand, lower inter-network connectivities including inter- DMN and FPN, frontal and temporal network (FTN) were observed due to possible neural source shifting and deactivation. Higher intra- and inter- FPN, VN, FTN, VN-DMN and SN network connectivities in counting condition compared to music and memory tasks were discovered, consistent with the hyper-connectivity of IPS/SFG/DLPFC VMHC values. Finally, as expected, more connection of intra- and inter- temporal, DMN-FPN, FTN and thalamocortical circuit were present during episodic memory recall condition. The dFNC connectogram confirmed the higher temporal dynamics of six representative networks such as higher DMN-CEN-MN connections at three task conditions compared to resting state. Small-worldness analysis revealed slightly higher global but lower local efficiencies in counting and music conditions together with relatively higher small-worldness weighting factor in the memory condition compared to resting state. Our multimodal neuroimaging results were consistent with published findings for each separate condition, and provided extra imaging evidence of arts and science training-related neuroplasticity and dynamic modulation enhancement of brain structure and function.

Keywords: dual regression, voxel-mirrored homotopic correlation, interhemispheric conductivity, functional specialization, efficiency, graph theory, small-worldness, brain atrophy, voxel-based morphometry, gray matter atrophy, fractional amplitude of low frequency fluctuation, PET/MRI, music, counting, episodic memory, medial prefrontal cortex, inferior frontal gyrus, anterior cingulate cortex, insular, superior temporal gyrus, occipital lobe, thalamus, cerebellum, motor area, supplementary motor area, intra-parietal sulcus, superior frontal gyrus, frontoparietal network, frontotemporal network, hippocampus, parahippocampus, posterior cingulate, precuneus, dorsolateral prefrontal cortex, superior parietal lobe, arts, science, abacus-based mental calculation, wisdom

1. Introduction

1.1. Overview of Music in Brain

Brain science including topics of cognitive function such as music/creativity training and experience as well as science education including mathematical practice, learning and memory could be investigated with neuroimaging approaches that provide objective and *in vivo* evidence of associated neuroplasticity changes and help elucidate the underlying neural mechanism [1]. Music experience involving singing, listening, playing and professional improvisation activated several brain circuits such as networks of emotion relief and pleasure, reward from anticipation to consumption, language system such as comprehension and communication as well as motor function from planning to coordination. In details, brain regions of anterior cingulate cortex (ACC) and insula were activated for singing, together with superior temporal gyrus (STG) and supramarginal gyrus (SMG) that co-activated when playing cello [2]. Also singing and instrumental music engaged regions of STG, especially the anterior planum polare and large temporal regions along the superior temporal sulcus that were involved more in singing [3]. Furthermore, familiar music correlated strongly with superior frontal gyrus (SFG) and thalamic neural activity, attributing to mind response of anticipating melodic rhythms as well as harmonic progression and lyric episodes in familiar songs [4]. And it had been confirmed that the STG, together with the supplementary/premotor areas were music-selective aside from scrambled stimuli, and different than the speech-selective regions in the medial temporal gyrus [5]. The supplementary motor area (SMA) was important in musical representation and execution for professional musicians, and sensorimotor network was enhanced during music listening and expertise enjoying [6, 7].

This paragraph reviewed music influences on multiple brain circuits including motivation, emotion, pleasure, reward, attention and neuroplasticity. From the neurobiological perspective, orexin cell that was primarily located in brain hypothalamus regulated stress response and also played important role in motivation and reward cycle [8]. And it had recently been reported that orexin or oxytocin levels linked to human musicality with similar cognition and emotion effects such as relief and trust/empathy, in addition to therapeutic improvements [9]. Moreover, the fronto-limbic interaction, such as connectivity between ventromedial prefrontal cortex (vmPFC) and striatum, was sensitive to music appreciation during the cognitive and emotion processing in addition to the spectral and temporal alterations of original music [10]. Also it had been proposed that the fronto-limbic and frontotemporal connectivity increments might form the basis for musical reward including possible emotional pleasure and motivation [11]. The musical effects on pleasure, reward and motivational learning had further been studied at various extensive neural centers, including the insula, thalamus, ventral striatum, ACC and temporal cortex such as STG [12-14]. Longitudinally, it had been reported that the insula, striatum and inferior frontal gyrus (IFG) activations increased over time during musical stimulus, possibly relating to long-term arts persistence and neuroplasticity exercises [15]. Brain local and global efficiencies including motor-auditory, executive and default mode networks (DMN) also presented alterations with different musical beats [16]. In addition, the structural connectivity from orbitofrontal cortex (OFC) (e.g., with striatum) was found to correlate with the music reward sensitivity individually [17]. Finally, connectivity between the insula and ACC network was increased in musicians and artists, resulting in better affective and empathic abilities as well as facilitative targeting attention (such as increased ACC activation in response to happy music) [18, 19].

1.2. Overview of Mathematics in Brain

The intra-parietal sulcus (IPS) maps numerical symbols and corresponding quantities in order for educated person to perform number-based mathematical operation, an analog to the cytoarchitectonic reference and structural-functional link in modern connectome [20, 21]. It had been discovered for a long time that IPS played important role in basic number representation and numerical development, even early in evolution [22-24]. Different magnitude shared similar activation patterns in the IPS based on neuroimaging findings, although some other distinct magnitude mechanism might exist [25]. In children, higher left IPS activity corresponded to better arithmetic scores; while IPS disorganization in early numerical development might cause lifelong arithmetic impairment [26, 27]. Also both counting and subitizing activated common network of IPS and middle occipital area [28]. And it was validated that professional mathematical reflection utilized IPS and ventral temporal region for elementary number sense [29].

In addition to IPS, prefrontal cortex (PFC) was used for mental calculation of numbers, and higher PFC activity was recruited for mathematical reasoning studies [30, 31]. Higher school grades such as 3rd grade compared to 2nd year had more PFC activation and hyper-connectivity between PFC and posterior brain regions [32]. One specific area, ACC, showed greater activation during the counting Stroop interference task, as well as increased connectivity with other frontal area during error monitoring of possible incorrect trials [33, 34]. The IPS and PFC together was considered as the core brain operation network for advanced mathematics in professional mathematicians and math-specific experts as well as for abstract problem solving in mental arithmetic [35-37]. The activity in the frontoparietal network (FPN) corresponded to numerical magnitude processing, and was the neural source for multiple demand tasks such as music, working memory and arithmetic [38, 39]. Finally, children showed higher diffused IPS and IFG frontoparietal activity with more attentional and processing efforts than concordant activity observed in adults during arithmetic processing in brain, especially during numerical fact retrieval that shared similar neural basis as phonological processing in brain [40].

1.3. Overview of Episodic Memory and Brain Imaging

Hippocampus served important role in re-experiencing episodic details from the recent, as well as activated for episodic condition in declarative memory [41, 42]. And it had been confirmed that the hippocampus, an important memory structure, was associated with the actual recollection of an event (episodic memory) [43]. The significant role of hippocampus and its seven main subfields, such as cornu ammonis (CA) subfield 1 (CA1), CA2, CA3, CA4, dentate gyrus (DG) and subiculum, in brain memory and cognitive function has been investigated extensively [44-46]. Specifically, the volumetry of each subfield, function of each division and modification at dementia disease status have been studied with advanced *in vivo* imaging technique recently, such as high field 7T MRI for high-resolution structural localization, and functional mapping with fast fMRI technique for memory encoding and retrieval [47-48]. The hippocampal abnormalities in early dementia such as mild cognitive impairment had been identified including CA3 and DG subfields for pattern discrimination, memory formation and encoding, retrieval and consolidation with advanced neuroimaging techniques (e.g., morphological shape and size, functional activity and connectivity metrics, and molecular imaging such as FDG-glucose metabolism, amyloid accumulation and tau deposition) [49-51]. Integrated simultaneous PET/MRI and multiparametric neuroimaging technique are the current trends that could pinpoint the actual memory process with more complementary profile and higher spatiotemporal resolution, and finally help improve the diagnosis accuracy and disease treatment [52, 53]. In addition, the cortical ventro-lateral prefrontal area demonstrated activations for working-memory process of spatial, verbal and visuospatial information; and these regions were consistently reported in episodic memory retrieval studies and validated in brain-damaged patients [54-56].

1.4. Objectives

Taken together, the training and practicing benefits of music such as singing, mathematics such as counting and episodic memory recall in brain had been summarized briefly. The purposes of this study are to: 1. investigate further specific brain imaging features including functional connectivity, conductivity, activity and synchrony, inter-network correlations and dynamic regulation of these task conditions in addition to conventional resting state with available fMRI data using multiple advanced quantitative imaging methods as in chapter 1; and 2. compare the statistical differences between each of two task conditions such as between music and counting tasks or between task and resting state condition to illustrate distinctive and relative alterations in brain under different states.

2. Methods and Data

2.1. Participants and Imaging Acquisitions

Imaging and phenotypic data were downloaded after approval from the website managed at the same NeuroImaging Tools & Resources Collaboratory (NITRC) database (www.nitrc.org) as in chapter 1. The fMRI dataset including structural and functional resting state as well as under three functional tasks were provided by the FIND lab (http://fcon_1000.projects.nitrc.org/indi/retro/find_stanford.html), as the INDI Prospective Data Sharing Samples hosted by NITRC (http://fcon_1000.projects.nitrc.org/indi/IndiPro.html). Three functional tasks were performed to the same participant together with the resting state acquisition using the counterbalanced order to study brain cognitive states [57]. These four conditions during each individual fMRI scan are listed as:

a. Resting state: Subjects were asked to relax with eyes closed.

b. Music: Subjects were asked to sing their favorite songs in their heads.

c. Counting by subtraction: Subjects were asked to count backwards from 5000 by 3s.

d. Episodic memory: Subjects were asked to recall the events of the day, from the time when they awoke until the last minute before they lay down in the scanner.

Thirteen participants including 8 women and 5 men, age range of 18-29 years with average of 24.1±1.0 years old, were enrolled in this study. MRI experiments were performed using the 3T MRI scanner with standardized imaging protocols. The 3D MPRAGE sequence was run with matrix size=512 x 512 x 176, resolution=0.47 x 0.47 x 0.9 mm^3. For the resting-state (RS) and three task fMRI data acquired for each individual, same imaging protocol was applied with standard gradient-echo EPI sequence (TR/TE=2000/30 msec, flip angle=80°, number of volumes=300, spatial resolution=3.4 x 3.4 x 4.5 mm^3) and total scan time of 10 minutes for each condition.

2.2. Imaging Parameters and Post-Processing

Similar MRI and fMRI image processing algorithms as in chapter 1 were implemented with the in-house developed scripts, to derive the conventional VMHC, VBM, ICA-DR, resting-state functional connectivity (RSFC) and fractional ALFF (fALFF) maps, as described in details in our previous works [8, 44, 58]. Typical and novel dynamic dFNC connectogram as well as regional homogeneity (ReHo) map together with small-worldness analyses were performed to all the four conditions. The details of data processing were introduced previously and outlined in our recently published works [59-60].

Voxel-wise between-group comparisons including VMHC and ICA-DR together with global mean statistical quantification including fALFF and small-worldness parameters were implemented among four conditions, such as between memory and resting-state, between music and counting conditions with both paired t-test and post-hoc statistical analysis.

3. Results

VMHC differences between each of three task conditions and resting state are demonstrated in Figure 1 for music, counting and memory respectively. VMHC reduction under music task condition (singing songs) compared to resting state (P<0.001) were mainly present in the visual, temporal, somatosensory and motor areas (Figure 1A). VMHC reduction under mathematical counting condition compared to resting state were found in similar regions as under music condition, but including more parietal regions with larger spatial spreading (Figure 1B). In Figure 1C, VMHC reduction under the episodic memory recall condition compared to resting state were observed in similar regions as to music condition, with slightly less statistical significance. The reductions of VMHC values in these task conditions were possibly due to the functional specialization of these regions for high-level cognitive process during expertise and science training, in contrast to the high inter-hemispheric correlation at resting state such as somatosensory/motor and occipital regions. For instance, the distinguishable activation only in IPS and SFG during counting task compared to resting state (deactivation of these regions) seemed to validate this hypothesis.

Differences between each of two task conditions including between music and memory, between counting and memory, between music and counting conditions were illustrated in Figure 2 (all with P<0.01). Compared to memory task, music task activated more in the medial and dorsolateral prefrontal cortices, anterior cingulate, striatum, superior temporal, occipital and cerebellum regions with higher VMHC values (Figure 2A). In contrast, the memory-related structure such as temporal cortex, posterior cingulate, frontal pole and parietal regions had higher conductivity at memory task compared to music condition. Moreover, frontoparietal regions including the intra-parietal sulcus and medial frontal region had higher VMHC at counting task compared to memory recall. Large areas of memory structure such as hippocampus, posterior cingulate, temporal lobe, DLPFC, visual cortex, somatomotor, parietal, thalamus, insular regions and basal ganglia demonstrated higher VMHC values at memory condition compared to counting condition (Figure 2B). Finally, Figure 2C showed higher VMHC values in the motor area/SMA, small clusters in the superior temporal segment, insular, visual cortex, amygdala, thalamus and anterior cingulate in music condition compared to counting situation. Similar to the counting-memory comparison, frontoparietal clusters, especially the intra-parietal sulcus and medial frontal region had higher VMHC at counting task condition compared to music task.

Figure 3 illustrated the intra- and inters- network connectivity differences with ICA-DR algorithm comparing singing song condition to resting state. Higher connectivities of frontal-parietal (FPN), default mode network (DMN), thalamo-temporal, fronto-visual, inter- salience (SN) and DMN were observed during music singing task compared to resting state (Figure 3, $P<0.01$). Furthermore, higher inter-network connectivities of SN-DMN, DMN-CEN, FPN, visuo-motor, temporal-DMN and frontal-DMN were found in the counting condition compared to resting state (Figure 4). Inter-network connectivity differences between memory and resting state in Figure 5 showed similar results as to counting comparison results in Figure 4, all with $P<0.01$.

Regarding the between-condition ICA-DR comparisons, Figure 6 identified higher frontal-DMN, thalamocortical, DMN-motor, frontal-SN and temporal-FPN connectivities together with lower inter-network connectivities of DMN-FPN, SN-DMN, fronto-temporal and fronto-visual circuits comparing music to counting conditions (P<0.01). Higher inter- and intra- DMN, SN-parietal, temporo-occipital, frontal and FPN connectivities were found in music condition compared to memory recall task; however, lower connectivities of FPN-DMN, frontotemporal, SN-temporal, thalamo-frontal, visual-DMN and motor-SN existed (Figure 7). Finally, ICA-DR differences comparing counting to memory conditions demonstrated higher network connectivities of intra- and inter- DMN, visual, thalamo-parietal, temporal and posterior FPN, DN-DMN and MN-FPN in counting condition compared to memory task (Figure 8). On the other hand, lower inter- DMN-FPN, temporal-FPN and thalamo-temporal connectivities existed comparing counting to memory conditions.

Using dFNC analysis, Figure 9 demonstrated the connectogram of a representative state (S3) for four conditions. Strong dynamic connections of DMN-CEN in music, DMN-MN in counting, DMN-MN/VN/CEN in memory and DMN-SN in resting conditions were observed. Overall, higher temporal dynamics at task conditions compared to resting state were observed, especially in the counting and music conditions (Figure 10). And longer mean dwell time in majorities of states were found under counting condition compared to three other conditions, possibly due to more active and attentional requirement of this specific task. Figure 11 presented similar distributions of mean dwell time distribution under both memory and resting state conditions. Lower mean dwell times were found under the music and memory conditions compared to resting state and counting condition, but no significant differences existed (Figure 12A). Relatively higher fractional frequencies in music and memory conditions were observed, but no significant differences among four conditions either (Figure 12B).

Slightly higher global but lower local efficiencies in counting and music conditions compared to resting state existed (Figure 13A). Relatively higher small-worldness factor in the memory condition compared to three other conditions were also observed (Figure 13B). Significantly lower VMHC (P=0.02) and fALFF (P<0.05, especially S5 and conventional bands) were found in three task conditions compared to resting state (Figure 14; P=0.046).

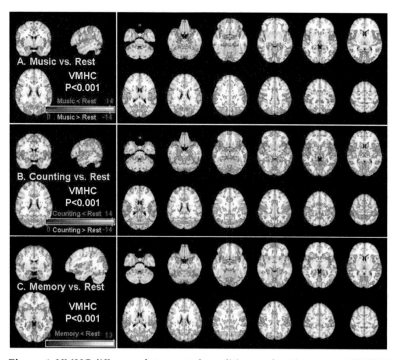

Figure 1. *VMHC differences between task conditions and resting state. A: VMHC reduction in music task condition (singing familiar songs) compared to resting state (P<0.001) in mainly the visual, somatosensory, motor areas, insular and small temporal clusters including the hippocampus. B: VMHC reduction in mathematical counting condition compared to resting state in similar regions as in*

A but including more parietal regions with wider spatial spreading; on the other hand, the intra-parietal sulcus and superior frontal region displayed higher VMHC during counting condition than resting state. C: VMHC reduction in the episodic memory recall condition compared to resting state in similar regions as to music condition as in A, including specific hippocampus and extra caudate regions.

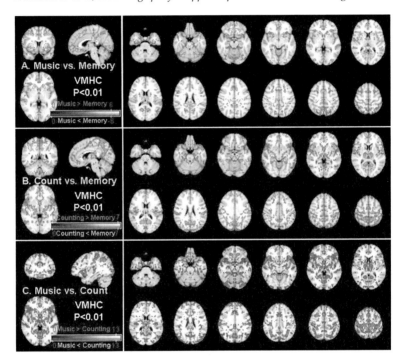

Figure 2. *Differences between each of two task conditions such as between music and memory (A), between counting and memory (B), as well as between music and counting conditions (C). For instance, panel C of the differences between music and counting conditions showed higher VMHC values in the motor area/SMA, superior temporal segment, insular, visual cortex, amygdala, thalamus and anterior cingulate in music condition. On the other hand, frontal parietal clusters and medial frontal region, especially the intra-parietal sulcus and frontal pole area showed higher VMHC at counting task compared to music condition. And the memory-related structure such as temporal cortex, posterior cingulate, precuneus and parietal regions had higher conductivity during memory task compared to music and counting conditions.*

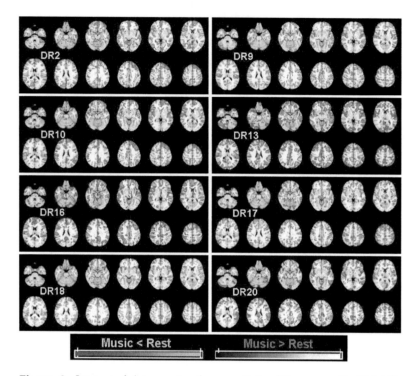

Figure 3. *Intra- and inter- network connectivity differences with ICA-DR algorithm comparing music singing condition to resting state. Higher connectivities of frontal-parietal, default mode network, thalamo-temporal fronto-visual, inter- salience and default mode networks were observed in music condition compared to resting state (P<0.01).*

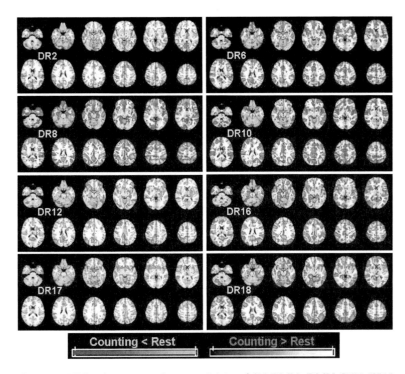

Figure 4. *Higher inter-network connectivities of SN-DMN, DMN-CEN, FPN, visuo-motor, temporal-DMN and frontal-DMN were found in the counting condition compared to resting state.*

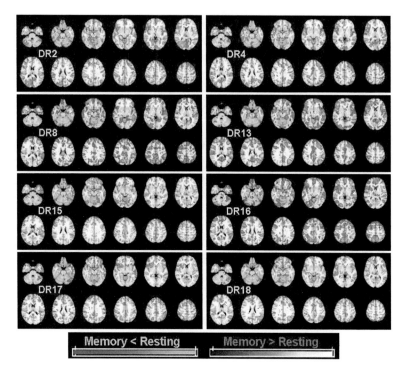

Figure 5. *Inter-network connectivity differences between memory and resting state showed similar results as to differences between counting and resting state as in Figure 3.*

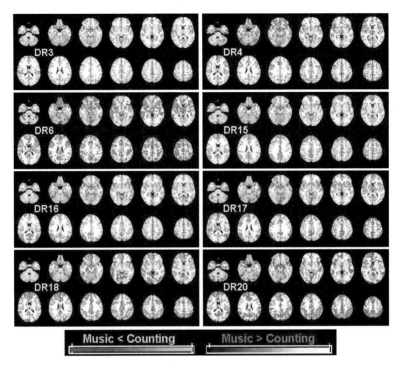

Figure 6. *Higher inter- frontal-DMN, thalamocortical, DMN-motor, frontal-SN, frontal-striatum and temporal-FPN network connectivities were found comparing music to counting conditions together with lower inter-network connectivities of DMN-FPN, SN-DMN, fronto-temporal and fronto-visual circuits (P<0.01).*

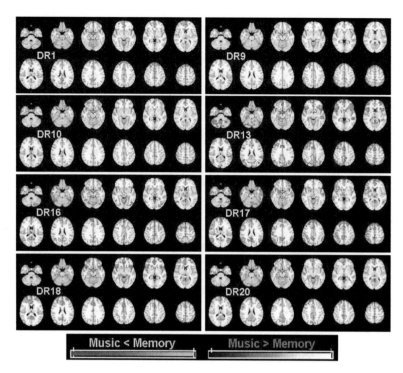

Figure 7. *Intra and inter-network connectivity differences between music and memory task conditions (P<0.01). Higher intra- and inter- DMN, SN-DMN, frontal, temporal, fronto-FPN connectivities were found at music task condition compared to memory task. On the other hand, higher network connectivities of frontal-thalamic, dorso-lateral prefrontal cortex (DLPFC)-DMN, frontotemporal, FPN-DMN, visual-DMN, temporal-SN circuits were identified at memory task compared to music condition as well.*

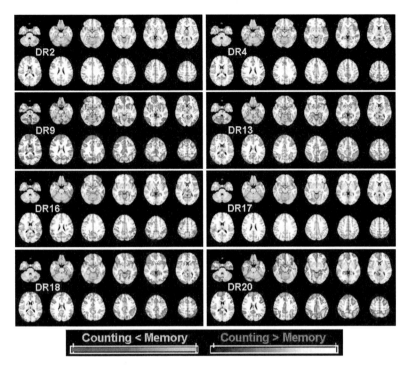

Figure 8. *Intra and inter-network connectivity differences between counting and memory task conditions (P<0.01). Higher intra- DMN, visual, thalamo-parietal, temporal and posterior FPN, SN-DMN and MN-FPN network connectivities in counting condition compared to memory task, together with lower inter- DMN-FPN, temporal-FPN, thalamo-temporal connectivities existed.*

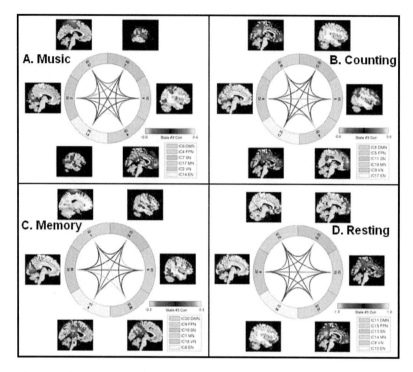

Figure 9. *Connectogram of a representative state (S3) of four conditions including panel A for music singing, B for mathematical counting, C for memory recall and D for resting state. Strong connections (dFNC) of DMN-CEN in music, DMN-MN in counting, DMN-MN/VN/CEN in memory and DMN-SN in resting conditions were observed.*

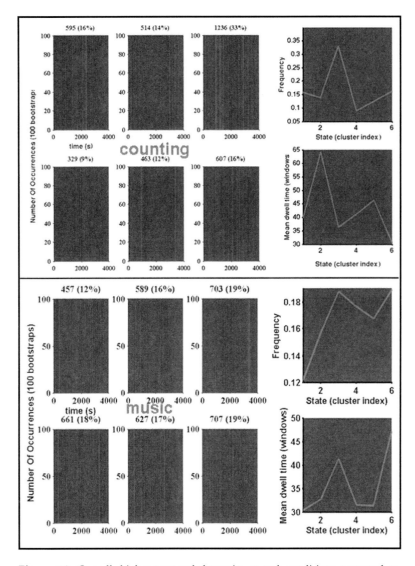

Figure 10. *Overall, higher temporal dynamics at task conditions compared to resting state were observed, especially in the counting and music conditions. And longer mean dwell time in majorities of states were found in counting condition compared to three other conditions, possibly due to more active and attentional requirement of this specific task.*

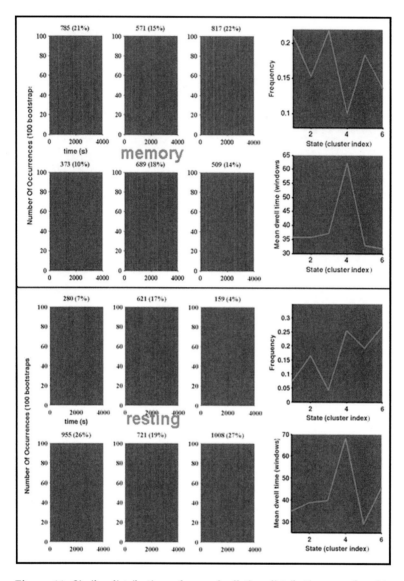

Figure 11. *Similar distributions of mean dwell time distribution were found in both memory and resting state condition.*

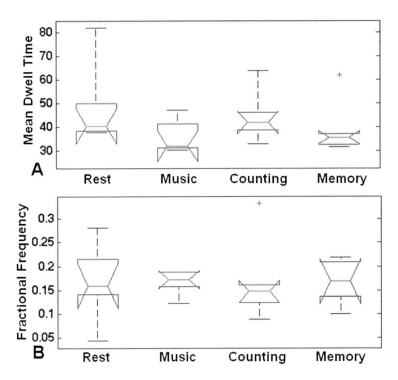

Figure 12. *A: Lower mean dwell times were found in the music and memory conditions compared to resting state and counting condition but no significant differences among four conditions. B: Relatively higher fractional frequencies in music and memory conditions and no significant differences between task and control conditions. The boxes have lines at the lower and upper quartile values (horizontal blue lines) as well as median (horizontal red lines) for the data in the column. The whiskers are lines extending from each end of the box to show the extent of the data, with the outliers plotted individually as the red cross sign.*

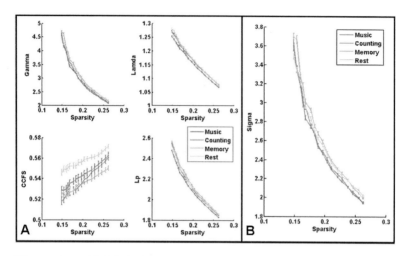

Figure 13. *A: Slightly higher global but lower local efficiencies in counting and music conditions compared to resting state; and B: relatively higher small-worldness factor in the memory condition compared to three other conditions were observed.*

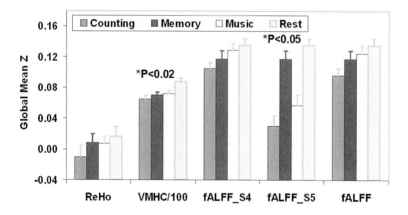

Figure 14. *Significantly lower global z-values of VMHC (P<0.02) and fALFF (especially sub-band S5 with P<0.05 and conventional band) were found in task conditions compared to resting state (P=0.046). Lower global ReHo and fALFF Z-values existed under three task conditions, but no significant differences were found among four conditions.*

4. Discussion

4.1. Summary of Results

In this study, we had performed all six conditional VMHC comparisons, including each of three task conditions in comparison to resting state, as well as between three-condition comparisons. Similar patterns with reduction of interhemispheric correlations in the visual, temporal, somatosensory and motor areas in music/counting/memory conditions compared to resting state were observed. The reductions of VMHC values in task condition were possibly due to the functional specialization of these regions at task condition, in contrast to the high inter-hemispheric correlation at resting state such as somatosensory/motor and occipital regions. Unique regional activation such as IPS and SFG during counting task condition compared to resting state (deactivation of these regions) and different spatial weighting of statistical significance in memory condition were revealed. Comparisons between each two of task conditions further demonstrated the distinct regional allocation of neural resources for each condition that imitated arts and science training program. Specifically, regions of medial prefrontal, anterior cingulate, insular, superior temporal, occipital, thalamus, cerebellum and motor/supplementary areas showed more interhemispheric correlations under singing songs condition, with larger differences comparing music to counting than memory recall tasks. The counting condition revealed more orbitofrontal interhemispheric correlation in addition to IPS and SFG compared to music/memory. And finally, clusters in the medial temporal lobe including hippocampus and parahippocampus, posterior cingulate, precuneus, DLPFC and superior parietal lobe maintained higher VMHC during episodic memory recall processing than music and counting tasks.

Functional connectivity based ICA-DR identified enhanced network connectivities of intra- DMN, FPN and SN during music singing condition compared to counting and memory recall tasks. On the other hand, lower inter-network connectivities including inter-DMN and FPN, frontotemporal network (FTN) were observed, possibly due to neural source shifting and deactivation. Higher intra- and inter- FPN, visual, FTN, VN-DMN and SN network connectivities in counting condition compared to music and memory tasks were discovered, consistent with the VMHC hyper-connectivity findings of IPS/SFG/DLPFC for mathematical operation. Finally, as expected, more connection of intra- and inter-temporal, DMN-FPN, FTN and thalamo-cortical networks were present during episodic memory recall condition.

The dFNC connectogram confirmed the higher temporal dynamics of six representative networks at task conditions compared to resting state, such as higher DMN-CEN-MN connections. And counting condition had longer mean dwell time in majorities of states than three other conditions, possibly due to more active and attentional requirement of this specific task. While global quantification identified relatively higher fractional frequencies in music and memory with relatively lower mean dwell times compared to counting and resting state. Small-worldness analysis revealed slightly higher global but lower local efficiencies in counting and music conditions together with relatively higher small-worldness weighting factor in the memory condition compared to resting state. Also global mean VMHC and fALFF including sub-band S5 values were significantly lower in three task conditions compared to resting conditions, indicating less global neural activity and circuits rerouting utilized in low frequency band in these tasks.

4.2. Comparison with Previous Findings

4.2.1. Music and Neuroplasticity

Brain has great capacity for new connections and optimistic pathways, while modern neuroimaging techniques enable functional studies related to professional scientific training and artistic performances. For instance, music listening could improve cognition and motor skills, and help brain recover after injury with music therapy as reported by many studies [61]. Right hemisphere was assumed to be associated more with music skill, performance coordination and three-dimensional visuospatial orientation; and particularly for perceiving pitch, melody, harmony and rhythm while sound frequency and intensity occurred more in the left hemisphere [62]. Specifically, the neural activity increased in several regions such as right STG, insular and IFG corresponding to complex tones for musicians compared to non-musicians [63]. During music practicing and training, structural volume changes of multiple brain regions and circuits including the posterior cingulate, insula and medial orbitofrontal cortex were exhibited [64]. These regions played important roles in executive function, memory, language and emotion regulation, and were consistent with our VMHC findings. A few typical large-scale networks showed stronger functional connectivity at resting state in professional musicians with more years of experience, including the SN, CEN, FTN and MN [65]. And several brain networks were recruited during musical creation such as DMN, CEN and MN in addition to SN for possible connection with STG [66]. Regional function specialization of music hierarchies had been suggested; for instance, STG was activated during melodic generation phase, while hippocampus and IFG for unexpected melodic sequences processing and FPN for possible violation prevention [67]. Furthermore, drum training induced long-term neuroplasticity change in the cerebellum such as larger gray matter volume in the left VIIIa section, together with cortical thickness increment in the left paracentral and right precuneus as part of cerebellar-cortical pathway [68]. Finally, the inter-network connectivities between VN and DMN, VN and CEN, DMN and CEN were higher in improvisational musicians but higher functional connectivities between DMN and frontal pole for classical musicians, and both having more intra- DMN and CEN connectivities as well as higher local and global efficiencies than controls [69].

Early training in life also has effective impact on the striatal-cortical-sensorimotor network for greater motor timing expertise; and music's neuroplasticity enhancement during fetal to infants had been emphasized [70, 71]. Furthermore, musical training increased functional connectivity of sensorimotor network together with higher structural connectivity of the auditory-motor network; and both related to practice time in young adults [72, 73]. Also structural deformation-based morphometry analyses demonstrated gray matter density change in the ventral premotor cortex (vPMC), and correlated with auditory motor synchronization performance as well as with age that reached highest plasticity at age range of 6-9 years old [74]. Moreover, singing modulated the experience-dependent vocal-motor control in the right anterior insular and sensorimotor areas, and involved heteromodal sensory/motor processing and interaction [75, 76]. In musicians and dancers, complex motor coordination integrated multimodal processing including not only the sensorimotor system such as the primary and secondary sensory/motor areas, but also the lateral PFC and IPS for necessary whole-body coordination and control [77].

4.2.2. Mental Mathematical Training and Neuroplasticity

In addition to IPS, a few other regions had been implicated consistently in arithmetic problem solving and mental calculation; including the left angular gyrus activation for retrieval of arithmetic facts and knowledge mostly, as well as the left superior frontoparietal region (such as gray matter density) for mathematical expertise and better performance [78, 79]. The rostrolateral PFC (rlPFC) had higher ReHo imaging values in children trained with abacus-based mental calculation (AMC) program compared to non-trained group, and tightly linked with improved inductive reasoning performance in these children [80]. Enhanced activation in the frontoparietal network (FPN) and visual cortex in the AMC group (in children especially) correlated with the arithmetical ability and visuospatial working memory (VSWM) neuroplasticity, a rapidly expanding developmental and cognitive science research field [81, 82]. Further AMC studies showed that enhanced bilateral superior parietal lobular functional coupling could lead to increased sustained FPN connectivity, through transferring effect to improve short-term working memory capacity [83, 84]. A few studies had validated improvement of cognitive/memory function and brain neural network with AMC training, including enhanced functional/anatomical FPN and occipitotemporal activation as well as increased micro-structural integrity in additional premotor areas [85, 86]. The association between neural plasticity in general training and cognitive improvements were further reported in trained young person with induced neuroplasticity [87]. Another abacus study reported increased functional connectivity between SMA and IFG, facilitating functional integration of visuospatial-attentional circuitry and high-level cognitive coordination [88]. Finally, memory function and systematic neuroimaging findings were reviewed in our recent work including multi-modal imaging elucidation of memory encoding/consolidation pathway together with multiomic applications in early mild cognitive impairments with memory concerns [44, 59].

4.3. Conclusion

In conclusion, we had reported brain functional and structural specialization at different task conditions including music, counting and memory. Distinct regional allocation of cognitive processing and network rerouting in three conditions were identified, including medial prefrontal, anterior cingulate, insular, superior temporal, occipital, thalamus, cerebellum and motor/supplementary areas for music singing; intra-parietal sulcus, superior frontal and orbitofrontal cortices for mathematical counting, medial temporal lobe and dorsolateral prefrontal cortex for episodic memory recall. The dFNC connectogram confirmed the higher temporal dynamics of six representative networks and neural source shifting at task conditions compared to resting state, such as higher DMN-CEN-MN connections. Our results were consistent with published findings for each separate condition, and provided extra imaging evidence of possible arts and scientific training-related neuroplasticity and dynamic modulation enhancement in brain.

References

[1] Wu CL, Lin TJ, Chiou GL, Lee CY, Luan H, Tsai MJ, Potvin P, Tsai CC. A Systematic Review of MRI Neuroimaging for Education Research. Front Psychol. 2021 May 20;12:617599. doi: 10.3389/fpsyg.2021.617599. PMID: 34093308; PMCID: PMC8174785.

[2] Segado M, Zatorre RJ, Penhune VB. Effector-independent brain network for auditory-motor integration: fMRI evidence from singing and cello playing. Neuroimage. 2021 Aug 15;237:118128. doi: 10.1016/j.neuroimage.2021.118128. Epub 2021 May 12. PMID: 33989814.

[3] Whitehead JC, Armony JL. Singing in the brain: Neural representation of music and voice as revealed by fMRI. Hum Brain Mapp. 2018 Dec;39(12):4913-4924. doi: 10.1002/hbm.24333. Epub 2018 Aug 18. PMID: 30120854; PMCID: PMC6866591.

[4] Freitas C, Manzato E, Burini A, Taylor MJ, Lerch JP, Anagnostou E. Neural Correlates of Familiarity in Music Listening: A Systematic Review and a Neuroimaging Meta-Analysis. Front Neurosci. 2018 Oct 5;12:686. doi: 10.3389/fnins.2018.00686. PMID: 30344470; PMCID: PMC6183416.

[5] Angulo-Perkins A, Concha L. Discerning the functional networks behind processing of music and speech through human vocalizations. PLoS One. 2019 Oct 10;14(10):e0222796. doi: 10.1371/journal.pone.0222796. PMID: 31600231; PMCID: PMC6786620.

[6] de Aquino MPB, Verdejo-Román J, Pérez-García M, Pérez-García P. Different role of the supplementary motor area and the insula between musicians and non-musicians in a controlled musical creativity task. Sci Rep. 2019 Sep 10;9(1):13006. doi: 10.1038/s41598-019-49405-5. PMID: 31506553; PMCID: PMC6736976.

[7] Krishnan S, Lima CF, Evans S, Chen S, Guldner S, Yeff H, Manly T, Scott SK. Beatboxers and Guitarists Engage Sensorimotor Regions Selectively When Listening to the Instruments They can Play. Cereb Cortex. 2018 Nov 1;28(11):4063-4079. doi: 10.1093/cercor/bhy208. PMID: 30169831; PMCID: PMC6188551.

[8] Zhou Y. *Multiparametric Imaging in Neurodegenerative Disease.* Nova Science Publishers. 2019.

[9] Harvey AR. Links Between the Neurobiology of Oxytocin and Human Musicality. Front Hum Neurosci. 2020 Aug 26;14:350. doi: 10.3389/fnhum.2020.00350. PMID: 33005139; PMCID: PMC7479205.

[10] Kim SG, Mueller K, Lepsien J, Mildner T, Fritz TH. Brain networks underlying aesthetic appreciation as modulated by interaction of the spectral and temporal organisations of music. Sci Rep. 2019 Dec 19;9(1):19446. doi: 10.1038/s41598-019-55781-9. PMID: 31857651; PMCID: PMC6923468.

[11] Zatorre RJ, Salimpoor VN. From perception to pleasure: music and its neural substrates. Proc Natl Acad Sci U S A. 2013 Jun 18;110 Suppl 2(Suppl 2):10430-7. doi: 10.1073/pnas.1301228110. Epub 2013 Jun 10. PMID: 23754373; PMCID: PMC3690607.

[12] Shany O, Singer N, Gold BP, Jacoby N, Tarrasch R, Hendler T, Granot R. Surprise-related activation in the nucleus accumbens interacts with music-induced pleasantness. Soc Cogn Affect Neurosci. 2019 May 17;14(4):459-470. doi: 10.1093/scan/nsz019. PMID: 30892654; PMCID: PMC6523415.

[13] Gold BP, Mas-Herrero E, Zeighami Y, Benovoy M, Dagher A, Zatorre RJ. Musical reward prediction errors engage the nucleus accumbens and motivate learning. Proc Natl Acad Sci U S A. 2019 Feb 19;116(8):3310-3315. doi: 10.1073/pnas. 1809855116. Epub 2019 Feb 6. PMID: 30728301; PMCID: PMC6386687.

[14] Petrini K, Crabbe F, Sheridan C, Pollick FE. The music of your emotions: neural substrates involved in detection of emotional correspondence between auditory and visual music actions. PLoS One. 2011 Apr 29;6(4):e19165. doi: 10.1371/journal. pone.0019165. PMID: 21559468; PMCID: PMC3084768.

[15] Koelsch S, Fritz T, V Cramon DY, Müller K, Friederici AD. Investigating emotion with music: an fMRI study. Hum Brain Mapp. 2006 Mar;27(3):239-50. doi: 10.1002/hbm.20180. PMID: 16078183; PMCID: PMC6871371.

[16] Toiviainen P, Burunat I, Brattico E, Vuust P, Alluri V. The chrronnectome of musical beat. Neuroimage. 2020 Aug 1;216:116191. doi: 10.1016/j.neuroimage.2019.116191. Epub 2019 Sep 13. PMID: 31525500.

[17] Martínez-Molina N, Mas-Herrero E, Rodríguez-Fornells A, Zatorre RJ, Marco-Pallarés J. White Matter Microstructure Reflects Individual

Differences in Music Reward Sensitivity. J Neurosci. 2019 Jun 19;39(25):5018-5027. doi: 10.1523/JNEUROSCI.2020-18.2019. Epub 2019 Apr 18. PMID: 31000588; PMCID: PMC6670256.

[18] Gujing L, Hui H, Xin L, Lirong Z, Yutong Y, Guofeng Y, Jing L, Shulin Z, Lei Y, Cheng L, Dezhong Y. Increased Insular Connectivity and Enhanced Empathic Ability Associated with Dance/Music Training. Neural Plast. 2019 May 6;2019:9693109. doi: 10.1155/2019/9693109. PMID: 31198419; PMCID: PMC6526550.

[19] Mitterschiffthaler MT, Fu CH, Dalton JA, Andrew CM, Williams SC. A functional MRI study of happy and sad affective states induced by classical music. Hum Brain Mapp. 2007 Nov;28(11):1150-62. doi: 10.1002/hbm.20337. PMID: 17290372; PMCID: PMC6871455.

[20] Dehaene S. Origins of mathematical intuitions: the case of arithmetic. Ann N Y Acad Sci. 2009 Mar;1156:232-59. doi: 10.1111/j.1749-6632.2009.04469.x. PMID: 19338511.

[21] Amunts K, Zilles K. Advances in cytoarchitectonic mapping of the human cerebral cortex. Neuroimaging Clin N Am. 2001 May;11(2):151-69, vii. PMID: 11489732.

[22] Wang L, Li M, Yang T, Wang L, Zhou X. Mathematics Meets Science in the Brain. Cereb Cortex. 2021 Jul 9:bhab198. doi: 10.1093/cercor/bhab198. Epub ahead of print. PMID: 34247249.

[23] Eger E, Sterzer P, Russ MO, Giraud AL, Kleinschmidt A. A supramodal number representation in human intraparietal cortex. Neuron. 2003 Feb 20;37(4):719-25. doi: 10.1016/s0896-6273(03)00036-9. PMID: 12597867.

[24] Dehaene S, Cohen L. Cultural recycling of cortical maps. Neuron. 2007 Oct 25;56(2):384-98. doi: 10.1016/j.neuron.2007.10.004. PMID: 17964253.

[25] Cohen Kadosh R, Lammertyn J, Izard V. Are numbers special? An overview of chronometric, neuroimaging, developmental and comparative studies of magnitude representation. Prog Neurobiol. 2008 Feb;84(2):132-47. doi: 10.1016/j.pneurobio. 2007.11.001. Epub 2007 Nov 19. PMID: 18155348.

[26] Bugden S, Price GR, McLean DA, Ansari D. The role of the left intraparietal sulcus in the relationship between symbolic number processing and children's arithmetic competence. Dev Cogn Neurosci. 2012 Oct;2(4):448-57. doi: 10.1016/j. dcn.2012.04.001. Epub 2012 Apr 21. PMID: 22591861; PMCID: PMC7005765.

[27] Dehaene S, Molko N, Cohen L, Wilson AJ. Arithmetic and the brain. Curr Opin Neurobiol. 2004 Apr;14(2):218-24. doi: 10.1016/j.conb.2004.03.008. PMID: 15082328.

[28] Piazza M, Mechelli A, Butterworth B, Price CJ. Are subitizing and counting implemented as separate or functionally overlapping processes? Neuroimage. 2002 Feb;15(2):435-46. doi: 10.1006/nimg.2001.0980. PMID: 11798277.

[29] Amalric M, Dehaene S. Cortical circuits for mathematical knowledge: evidence for a major subdivision within the brain's semantic networks. Philos Trans R Soc Lond B Biol Sci. 2017 Feb 19;373(1740):20160515. doi: 10.1098/rstb.2016.0515. PMID: 29292362; PMCID: PMC5784042.

[30] Arsalidou M, Taylor MJ. Is 2+2=4? Meta-analyses of brain areas needed for numbers and calculations. Neuroimage. 2011 Feb 1;54(3):2382-93. doi: 10.1016/j.neuroimage.2010.10.009. Epub 2010 Oct 12. PMID: 20946958.

[31] Eliez S, Blasey CM, Menon V, White CD, Schmitt JE, Reiss AL. Functional brain imaging study of mathematical reasoning abilities in velocardiofacial syndrome (del22q11.2). Genet Med. 2001 Jan-Feb;3(1):49-55. doi: 10.1097/00125817-200101000-00011. PMID: 11339378.

[32] Rosenberg-Lee M, Barth M, Menon V. What difference does a year of schooling make? Maturation of brain response and connectivity between 2nd and 3rd grades during arithmetic problem solving. Neuroimage. 2011 Aug 1;57(3):796-808. doi: 10.1016/j.neuroimage.2011.05.013. Epub 2011 May 18. PMID: 21620984; PMCID: PMC3165021.

[33] Bush G, Whalen PJ, Rosen BR, Jenike MA, McInerney SC, Rauch SL. The counting Stroop: an interference task specialized for functional neuroimaging--validation study with functional MRI. Hum Brain Mapp. 1998;6(4):270-82. doi: 10.1002/(SICI)1097-0193(1998)6:4<270::AID-HBM6>3.0.CO;2-0. PMID: 9704265; PMCID: PMC6873370.

[34] Zhou X, Li M, Li L, Zhang Y, Cui J, Liu J, Chen C. The semantic system is involved in mathematical problem solving. Neuroimage. 2018 Feb 1;166:360-370. doi: 10.1016/j.neuroimage.2017.11.017. Epub 2017 Nov 10. PMID: 29129671.

[35] Amalric M, Dehaene S. Origins of the brain networks for advanced mathematics in expert mathematicians. Proc Natl Acad Sci U S A. 2016 May 3;113(18):4909-17. doi: 10.1073/pnas.1603205113. Epub 2016 Apr 11. PMID: 27071124; PMCID: PMC4983814.

[36] Emerson RW, Cantlon JF. Early math achievement and functional connectivity in the fronto-parietal network. Dev Cogn Neurosci. 2012 Feb 15;2 Suppl 1(Suppl 1):S139-51. doi: 10.1016/j.dcn.2011.11.003. Epub 2011 Nov 22. Erratum in: Dev Cogn Neurosci. 2012 Apr;2(2):291. PMID: 22682903; PMCID: PMC3375498.

[37] Tschentscher N, Hauk O. How are things adding up? Neural differences between arithmetic operations are due to general problem solving strategies. Neuroimage. 2014 May 15;92:369-80. doi: 10.1016/j.neuroimage.2014.01.061. Epub 2014 Feb 10. PMID: 24525170.

[38] Wilkey ED, Price GR. Attention to number: The convergence of numerical magnitude processing, attention, and mathematics in the inferior frontal gyrus. Hum Brain Mapp. 2019 Feb 15;40(3):928-943. doi: 10.1002/hbm.24422. Epub 2018 Nov 2. PMID: 30387895; PMCID: PMC6615546.

[39] Mineroff Z, Blank IA, Mahowald K, Fedorenko E. A robust dissociation among the language, multiple demand, and default mode networks: Evidence from inter-region correlations in effect size. Neuropsychologia. 2018 Oct;119:501-511. doi: 10.1016/j.neuropsychologia.2018.09.011. Epub 2018 Sep 20. PMID: 30243926; PMCID: PMC6191329..

[40] Pollack C, Ashby NC. Where arithmetic and phonology meet: The meta-analytic convergence of arithmetic and phonological processing in the brain. Dev Cogn Neurosci. 2018 Apr;30:251-264. doi: 10.1016/j.dcn.2017.05.003. Epub 2017 May 10. PMID: 28533112; PMCID: PMC6969128.

[41] Piolino P, Desgranges B, Eustache F. Episodic autobiographical memories over the course of time: cognitive, neuro-psychological and neuroimaging findings. Neuropsychologia. 2009 Sep;47(11):2314-29. doi: 10.1016/j.neuropsychologia.2009.01.020. Epub 2009 Jan 19. PMID: 19524095.

[42] Cabeza R, Nyberg L. Functional neuroimaging of memory. Neuropsychologia. 2003;41(3):241-4. doi: 10.1016/s0028-3932(02)00156-2. PMID: 12457749.

[43] Schacter DL. The cognitive neuroscience of memory: perspectives from neuroimaging research. Philos Trans R Soc Lond B Biol Sci. 1997 Nov 29;352(1362):1689-95. doi: 10.1098/rstb.1997.0150. PMID: 9415920; PMCID: PMC1692095.

[44] Zhou Y. *Imaging and Multiomic Biomarker Applications: Advances in Early Alzheimer's Disease*. Nova Science Publishers. 2020.

[45] Yushkevich PA, Avants BB, Pluta J, et al. Shape-based alignment of hippocampal subfields: evaluation in postmortem MRI. Med Image Comput Assist Interv. 2008;11(1):510-7.

[46] Adler DH, Wisse LEM, Ittyerah R, et al. Characterizing the human hippocampus in aging and Alzheimer's disease using a computational atlas derived from ex vivo MRI and histology. Proc Natl Acad Sci U S A. 2018;115(16):4252-4257.

[47] Van Leemput K, Bakkour A, Benner T, Wiggins G, et al. Automated segmentation of hippocampal subfields from ultra-high resolution in vivo MRI. Hippocampus. 2009;19(6):549-57.

[48] Olsen RK, Carr VA, Daugherty AM, et al. Progress update from the hippocampal subfields group. Alzheimers Dement (Amst). 2019;11:439-449.

[49] Chen X, Zhou Y, Wang R, et al. Potential Clinical Value of Multiparametric PET in the Prediction of Alzheimer's Disease Progression. PLoS One. 2016;11(5):e0154406.

[50] Eliassen CF, Reinvang I, Selnes P, et al. Biomarkers in subtypes of mild cognitive impairment and subjective cognitive decline. Brain Behav. 2017;7(9):e00776.

[51] Choi EJ, Son YD, Noh Y, et al. Glucose Hypometabolism in Hippocampal Subdivisions in Alzheimer's Disease: A Pilot Study Using High-Resolution [18]

[52] Yan S, Zheng C, Cui B, et al. Multiparametric imaging hippocampal neurodegeneration and functional connectivity with simultaneous PET/MRI in Alzheimer's disease. Eur J Nucl Med Mol Imaging. 2020;47(10):2440-2452

[53] Carlson ML, DiGiacomo PS, Fan AP, et al. Simultaneous FDG-PET/MRI detects hippocampal subfield metabolic differences in AD/MCI. Sci Rep. 2020;10(1):12064.

[54] Owen AM. The role of the lateral frontal cortex in mnemonic processing: the contribution of functional neuroimaging. Exp Brain Res. 2000 Jul;133(1):33-43. doi: 10.1007/s002210000398. PMID: 10933208.

[55] Squire LR, Zola SM. Episodic memory, semantic memory, and amnesia. Hippocampus. 1998;8(3):205-11. doi: 10.1002/(SICI) 1098-1063(1998)8:3<205::AID-HIPO3>3.0.CO;2-I. PMID: 9662135.

[56] Platel H. Functional neuroimaging of semantic and episodic musical memory. Ann N Y Acad Sci. 2005 Dec;1060:136-47. doi: 10.1196/annals.1360.010. PMID: 16597760.

[57] Shirer WR, Ryali S, Rykhlevskaia E, Menon V, Greicius MD. Decoding subject-driven cognitive states with whole-brain connectivity patterns. Cereb Cortex. 2012 Jan;22(1):158-65. doi: 10.1093/cercor/ bhr099. Epub 2011 May 26. PMID: 21616982; PMCID: PMC3236795.

[58] Zhou Y. *Joint Imaging Applications in General Neurodegenerative Disease: Parkinson's, Frontotemporal, Vascular Dementia and Autism.* Nova Science Publishers. 2021.

[59] Zhou Y. *Functional Neuroimaging with Multiple Modalities: Principle, Device and Applications.* Nova Science Publishers. 2016.

[60] Zhou Y. *Typical Imaging in Atypical Parkinson's, Schizophrenia, Epilepsy and Asymptomatic Alzheimer's Disease.* Nova Science Publishers. 2021.

[61] Demarin V, Bedeković MR, Puretić MB, Pašić MB. Arts, Brain and Cognition. Psychiatr Danub. 2016 Dec;28(4):343-348. PMID: 27855424.

[62] Bosnar-Puretić M, Roje-Bedeković M, Demarin V. The art: neuroscientific approach. Acta Clin Croat. 2009 Sep;48(3):367-70. PMID: 20055265.

[63] Bianchi F, Hjortkjær J, Santurette S, Zatorre RJ, Siebner HR, Dau T. Subcortical and cortical correlates of pitch discrimination: Evidence for two levels of neuroplasticity in musicians. Neuroimage. 2017 Dec;163:398-412. doi: 10.1016/j.neuroimage.2017.07.057. Epub 2017 Jul 31. PMID: 28774646

[64] Chaddock-Heyman L, Loui P, Weng TB, Weisshappel R, McAuley E, Kramer AF. Musical Training and Brain Volume in Older Adults. Brain Sci. 2021 Jan 5;11(1):50. doi: 10.3390/brainsci11010050. PMID: 33466337; PMCID: PMC7824792.

[65] Zamorano AM, Cifre I, Montoya P, Riquelme I, Kleber B. Insula-based networks in professional musicians: Evidence for increased functional connectivity during resting state fMRI. Hum Brain Mapp. 2017

Oct;38(10):4834-4849. doi: 10.1002/hbm.23682. Epub 2017 Jul 24. PMID: 28737256; PMCID: PMC6866802.

[66] Bashwiner DM, Bacon DK, Wertz CJ, Flores RA, Chohan MO, Jung RE. Resting state functional connectivity underlying musical creativity. Neuroimage. 2020 Sep;218:116940. doi: 10.1016/j.neuroimage. 2020.116940. Epub 2020 May 15. PMID: 32422402.

[67] Martins MJD, Fischmeister FPS, Gingras B, Bianco R, Puig-Waldmueller E, Villringer A, Fitch WT, Beisteiner R. Recursive music elucidates neural mechanisms supporting the generation and detection of melodic hierarchies. Brain Struct Funct. 2020 Sep;225(7):1997-2015. doi: 10.1007/s00429-020-02105-7. Epub 2020 Jun 26. PMID: 32591927; PMCID: PMC7473971.

[68] Bruchhage MMK, Amad A, Draper SB, Seidman J, Lacerda L, Laguna PL, Lowry RG, Wheeler J, Robertson A, Dell'Acqua F, Smith MS, Williams SCR. Drum training induces long-term plasticity in the cerebellum and connected cortical thickness. Sci Rep. 2020 Jun 22;10(1):10116. doi: 10.1038/s41598-020-65877-2. PMID: 32572037; PMCID: PMC7308330.

[69] Belden A, Zeng T, Przysinda E, Anteraper SA, Whitfield-Gabrieli S, Loui P. Improvising at rest: Differentiating jazz and classical music training with resting state functional connectivity. Neuroimage. 2020 Feb 15;207:116384. doi: 10.1016/j.neuroimage.2019.116384. Epub 2019 Nov 21. PMID: 31760149.

[70] van Vugt FT, Hartmann K, Altenmüller E, Mohammadi B, Margulies DS. The impact of early musical training on striatal functional connectivity. Neuroimage. 2021 Sep;238:118251. doi: 10.1016/j.neuroimage.2021. 118251. Epub 2021 Jun 8. PMID: 34116147.

[71] Chorna O, Filippa M, De Almeida JS, Lordier L, Monaci MG, Hüppi P, Grandjean D, Guzzetta A. Neuroprocessing Mechanisms of Music during Fetal and Neonatal Develop-ment: A Role in Neuroplasticity and Neurodevelopment. Neural Plast. 2019 Mar 20;2019:3972918. doi: 10.1155/2019/3972918. PMID: 31015828; PMCID: PMC6446122.

[72] Li Q, Wang X, Wang S, Xie Y, Li X, Xie Y, Li S. Musical training induces functional and structural auditory-motor network plasticity in young adults. Hum Brain Mapp. 2018 May;39(5):2098-2110. doi: 10.1002/hbm.23989. Epub 2018 Feb 5. PMID: 29400420; PMCID: PMC6866316.

[73] Zuk J, Gaab N. Evaluating predisposition and training in shaping the musician's brain: the need for a developmental perspective. Ann N Y Acad Sci. 2018 May 24:10.1111/nyas.13737. doi: 10.1111/nyas.13737. Epub ahead of print. PMID: 29799116; PMCID: PMC6252158.

[74] Bailey JA, Zatorre RJ, Penhune VB. Early musical training is linked to gray matter structure in the ventral premotor cortex and auditory-motor rhythm synchronization performance. J Cogn Neurosci. 2014 Apr;26(4):755-67. doi: 10.1162/jocn_a_00527. Epub 2013 Nov 18. PMID: 24236696.

[75] Kleber B, Zeitouni AG, Friberg A, Zatorre RJ. Experience-dependent modulation of feedback integration during singing: role of the right anterior insula. J Neurosci. 2013 Apr 3;33(14):6070-80. doi: 10.1523/JNEUROSCI.4418-12.2013. PMID: 23554488; PMCID: PMC6618920.

[76] Zatorre RJ, Baum SR. Musical melody and speech intonation: singing a different tune. PLoS Biol. 2012;10(7):e1001372. doi: 10.1371/journal.pbio.1001372. Epub 2012 Jul 31. PMID: 22859909; PMCID: PMC3409119.

[77] Ladda AM, Wallwork SB, Lotze M. Multimodal Sensory-Spatial Integration and Retrieval of Trained Motor Patterns for Body Coordination in Musicians and Dancers. Front Psychol. 2020 Nov 17;11:576120. doi: 10.3389/fpsyg.2020.576120. PMID: 33312150; PMCID: PMC7704436.

[78] van Eimeren L, Grabner RH, Koschutnig K, Reishofer G, Ebner F, Ansari D. Structure-function relationships underlying calculation: a combined diffusion tensor imaging and fMRI study. Neuroimage. 2010 Aug 1;52(1):358-63. doi: 10.1016/j.neuroimage.2010.04.001. Epub 2010 Apr 9. PMID: 20382234.

[79] Popescu T, Sader E, Schaer M, Thomas A, Terhune DB, Dowker A, Mars RB, Cohen Kadosh R. The brain-structural correlates of mathematical expertise. Cortex. 2019 May;114:140-150. doi: 10.1016/j.cortex.2018.10.009. Epub 2018 Oct 22. PMID: 30424836; PMCID: PMC6996130.

[80] Jia X, Zhang Y, Yao Y, Chen F, Liang P. Neural correlates of improved inductive reasoning ability in abacus-trained children: A resting state fMRI study. Psych J. 2021 Aug;10(4):566-573. doi: 10.1002/pchj.439. Epub 2021 Mar 11. PMID: 33709543.

[81] Wang C, Xu T, Geng F, Hu Y, Wang Y, Liu H, Chen F. Training on Abacus-Based Mental Calculation Enhances Visuospatial Working Memory in Children. J Neurosci. 2019 Aug 14;39(33):6439-6448. doi: 10.1523/JNEUROSCI.3195-18.2019. Epub 2019 Jun 17. PMID: 31209171; PMCID: PMC6697396.

[82] Wang C, Geng F, Yao Y, Weng J, Hu Y, Chen F. Abacus Training Affects Math and Task Switching Abilities and Modulates Their Relationships in Chinese Children. PLoS One. 2015 Oct 7;10(10):e0139930. doi: 10.1371/journal.pone.0139930. PMID: 26444689; PMCID: PMC4596702.

[83] Zhou H, Geng F, Wang T, Wang C, Xie Y, Hu Y, Chen F. Training on Abacus-based Mental Calculation Enhances Resting State Functional Connectivity of Bilateral Superior Parietal Lobules. Neuroscience. 2020 Apr 15;432:115-125. doi: 10.1016/j.neuroscience.2020.02.033. Epub 2020 Feb 27. PMID: 32112920.

[84] Zhou H, Geng F, Wang Y, Wang C, Hu Y, Chen F. Transfer effects of abacus training on transient and sustained brain activation in the frontal-parietal network. Neuroscience. 2019 Jun 1;408:135-146. doi: 10.1016/j.neuroscience.2019.04.001. Epub 2019 Apr 11. PMID: 30981864.

[85] Wang C. A Review of the Effects of Abacus Training on Cognitive Functions and Neural Systems in Humans. Front Neurosci. 2020 Sep 2;14:913. doi: 10.3389/fnins.2020.00913. PMID: 32982681; PMCID: PMC7492585.

[86] Hu Y, Geng F, Tao L, Hu N, Du F, Fu K, Chen F. Enhanced white matter tracts integrity in children with abacus training. Hum Brain Mapp. 2011 Jan;32(1):10-21. doi: 10.1002/hbm.20996. PMID: 20235096; PMCID: PMC6870462.

[87] Tymofiyeva O, Gaschler R. Training-Induced Neural Plasticity in Youth: A Systematic Review of Structural and Functional MRI Studies. Front Hum Neurosci. 2021 Jan 18;14:497245. doi: 10.3389/fnhum.2020.497245. PMID: 33536885; PMCID: PMC7848153.

[88] Li Y, Hu Y, Zhao M, Wang Y, Huang J, Chen F. The neural pathway underlying a numerical working memory task in abacus-trained children and associated functional connectivity in the resting brain. Brain Res. 2013 Nov 20;1539:24-33. doi: 10.1016/j.brainres.2013.09.030. Epub 2013 Sep 28. PMID: 24080400.

Chapter 3
Structural and Functional Neuroimaging Correlates of Emotion, Intelligence and Wisdom

Abstract

The objectives of this chapter were to investigate the brain changes such as neural activity and myelin-related functional correlation as well as morphological/ microstructural connectivity-based neuroplasticity improvements during college training with baseline and longitudinal imaging and phenotypic data. For the fALFF correlational results, several regions presented significantly positive correlations between fALFF neural activities and four aspects of emotional intelligence (EI) scores including insula, hypothalamus, cuneus and motor areas at all three time points. Longitudinally, increased associations between fALFF and EI scores were observed in the visuospatial regions and frontal medial/dorso-lateral portions. For trait association, fALFF neural activities in some similar regions such as frontal, motor/supplementary motor areas, thalamus, basal ganglia and temporoparietal regions also presented negative association with different aspects of the trait scores at three time points. For the ReHo associations, EI scores including all four aspects were positively associated with regional homogeneity in the parietal/superior temporal cluster and premotor/motor areas. During all the three time points, Raven's CRT score was positively associated with ReHo values in the orbitofrontal and superior frontal, insular, superior temporal and motor/supplementary motor area. For the VMHC, significant longitudinal VMHC increments in the inferior temporal area, posterior cingulate and inferior parietal regions were observed. VMHC values in the cerebellum, temporal cortex including hippocampus/parahippocampus and superior segment, sensorimotor area and occipital/parietal lobes showed consistently negative associations with the depression/anxiety scores.

Significant positive correlations between gray matter density in the cerebellum, insular, orbitofrontal, fusiform, cuneus, posterior cingulate, medial prefrontal, subcortical caudate and putamen regions were observed with the EI scores of four domains including appraisal, monitoring, social ability and utilization at three time points. While cortical temporal regions including hippocampus and parahippocampus, orbitofrontal and superior frontal, visual and sensorimotor areas demonstrated significant correlations and predictions with depression and trait/state anxiety scores mainly. Associations between EI/trait scores and DTI FA/diffusivities in several tracts of the thalamic radiation, splenium of corpus callosum, internal capsule, cingulum, superior longitudinal fasciculus and cortico-spinal tract were identified at all time points. Finally, significantly increased global and decreased local efficiencies longitudinally were identified, indicating a more optimal and efficient brain network topology at later time point after college training. In line with the results presented in previous Chapters 1 and 2, these brain regions showed improvements of neural activity, synchrony and integration, myelin-related conductivity, morphological and microstructural connectivity for better performance and achievement with skills training, emotional and social interaction as well as knowledge accumulation.

Keywords: neuroplasticity, neurodevelopment, education, college life, longitudinal analysis, emotional intelligence, trait, anxiety, depression, combined Raven's test, insular, orbitofrontal cortex, fusiform, cuneus, posterior cingulate, medial prefrontal cortex, social ability, diffusion tensor imaging, correlational test, phenotypic association, arts, science

1. Introduction

For well education, college life cultivates professional skills, improves social interaction and communication, broadens vision and expands mind, gains experience and expertise, and finally enriches knowledge and creativity. Emotional intelligence (EI) and general intelligence that were used for reasoning and analyzing to solve problems are usually emphasized for improvement during academic training. People with normal and high intelligence, especially superior EI ability, could perform better in complicate environment and obtain more academic achievement with successful appraisal, monitoring and utilization of emotions and social skills [1]. Also positive effects of emotional regulation and facilitation in after-college life had showed promotions of creativity and mood with better working environment as well as enhanced interpersonal communication with excellent EI. In contrast, abnormal and deficient EI might lead to negative emotions, primarily depression and anxiety (both state and trait) that could affect life-time quality without proper handling and cure [2]. In the brain, neural correlates of emotion and intelligence had been studied extensively and remained as one of the most active research and educational fields. Imaging findings regarding different aspects of EI such as utilization/appraisal and their corresponding activations, cortical attachment of general intelligence and anxiety/depression traits will be reviewed in this section. General introduction of related specific results from the data used in this chapter and what remains to be discovered will be outlined in the end, with the hope to present another structural and functional neuroimaging application example in the educational and neurodevelopmental research area [3-6].

Several gray matter structures had been associated with different EI aspects based on MRI voxel-wise morphometry for gray matter density (GMD) and gray matter volume (GMV) quantifications [7]. For instance, insular and orbitofrontal GMD correlated with monitor of emotions, parahippocampal GMV correlated with utilization of EI, and cerebellar vermis GMV related to social ability. GMVs of the supplementary motor area (SMA) and anterior cingulate cortex (ACC) were negatively associated with artistic creativity, while GMVs of medial prefrontal cortex (MPFC) and inferior occipital gyrus (IOG) were positively associated with scientific creativity [8]. And it had further been validated that the GMV of premotor cortex

(PMC) had significant positive correlation with the creative achievement and art scores, a region responsible for novel action creation and decision selection as well as motor inhibition that might be changed with training and practice with neuroplasticity characteristics [9]. Higher correlation slopes between ACC/MPFC and creative score measured with figural Torrance test of Creative thinking (TTCT-F) were reported in college students with art majors than non-art majors [10]. GMV and white matter volume (WMV) of another typical region, inferior frontal gyrus (IFG), were significantly related to the verbal creativity ability, and IFG was crucial for language production and comprehension as well as representation/expression [11]. And finally in the dorsolateral prefrontal cortex (DLPFC), link between GMV and visuospatial ability measured with Raven's Matrices reasoning capacity was greater in males than in females; while females had larger IFG GMV-verbal reasoning ability correlation and higher MPFC GMV-information binding score than males [12]. GMV of DLPFC together with ACC and ventral striatum (VST) were associated with self-monitoring score [13]. Lastly, brain activity differed between adolescents and adults (i.e., aging effects) with distinct activity patterns in ACC and ventromedial prefrontal cortex (vmPFC) for attention and decision making, but not in VST [14]. The VST, on the other hand, functionally coupled to the IFG/insular and orbitofrontal cortex, changed connectivity according to the emotional context during inhibitory control [15].

Furthermore, based on large scale connectome of effective causality analysis, effective connectivity of central executive network (CEN) and salience network (SN) played important roles in regulating and processing emotions that might serve as biomarker for EI neural mechanism [16]. And as reported previously, structural morphology of SN was involved in artistic creativity, while CEN and semantic processing was highly related to scientific innovation [8]. The superior parietal lobe was linked to the EI as node of network topology for default mode network (DMN) in high EI scoring individuals, and possible the dorsal attentional network (DAN) in lower-score subjects [17]. Functional connectivity of vmPFC correlated with EI scores in depressed people, with reduced connectivity between anterior medial frontal and cingulate regions [18]. Moreover, GMV of parahippocampal gyrus (PHG) and fusiform together with the WMV of the superior temporal gyrus (STG) in right hemisphere were related to the depression severity measured with automatic thoughts questionnaire (ATQ) in preclinical depressed individuals [19]. In addition, the GMV of PHG correlated with ATQ score, and negative ATQ mediated correlation between PHG GMV and depression scale [20].

Some intra- and inter-network metrics such as within the MPFC-precuneus resting-state functional connectivity (RSFC) were negatively correlated to the creativity score; however, positive relationship was discovered between left-right DLPFC RSFC and creativity scale [21]. The increased within-DMN and MPFC-medial temporal gyrus (MTG) RSFC contributed to the creativity after training of cognitive stimulation, reflecting creativity training-induced changes in functional connectivity, especially in the low creativity individuals who had worse scores of TTCT [22]. Microstructural integrity measure such as fractional anisotropy (FA) with MRI diffusion tensor imaging (DTI) found FAs of superior longitudinal fasciculus and cortico-spinal tract were associated with EI appraisal score, and structural integrity of major forceps/uncinate fasciculus related to EI monitoring and managing [23]. FA of the anterior cingulum correlated negatively with self-monitoring score, and FA in the inferior parietal lobe and STG correlated with empathizing quotient (EQ) in females with opposite effects in males [13, 24]. After controlling for age and gender, FA values of several tracts including inferior fronto-occipital fasciculus and uncinate fasciculus that linked to broad cortical networks, were correlated negatively with composite creative index consistently in a large data cohort [25].

Results of other metrics such as regional coherence (ReHo) had been reported including positive correlation between ReHo of frontoparietal network (FPN) and intelligence, in addition to the multiple lower network-complexities of motor, attention, emotion, CEN and DMN for elderly adults [26, 27]. And ReHo within the DMN system reflecting synchronous activities, correlated with the perceived social support [28]. The intrinsic neural activity measured with fractional amplitude of low frequency fluctuation (fALFF) and ReHo values in the expected vmPFC and ACC regions were significantly associated with the trait anxiety, while changes of neural activity predicted state anxiety score variability over 9-month interval [29]. Correlation between ALFF neural activity and negative affectivity were different between depressed and control groups, and higher MPFC ALFF might be a resilience biomarker to depression in the elderly adults. On the other hand, lower neural activity in the regions of amygdala, vmPFC and posterior cingulate cortex (PCC) indicated successful emotion regulation in never-depressed individuals with high negative affection [30]. And amygdala was usually highlighted in individuals with mood disorder, together with lower activity in ACC/parietal cortex for emotional regulation that indicated attentional allocation deficits of anxiety disorder [31]. Also reflective wisdom might contribute to the healthier ego-identity formation as part of the social ability with significant correlations between two measures [32]. Biological factors including age and gender as well as educational level and social interactions influenced intelligence test results such as Mayer-Salovey-Caruso-Emotional-Intelligence-Test (MSCEIT) slightly, with higher education level and excellent social interactions correlating positively to EI [33, 34]. Moreover, it was generally accepted that main EI function and capability help protect against depression, especially for elderly adults [35]. And brain reserve, particularly the neuroplasticity gains over lifetime intellectual activities/experience, could preserve healthy cognitive-emotional structure at aging and remain less vulnerable to functional impairments of age-related diseases such as metabolic syndrome and dementia [36].

Investigation of full-spectrum intelligence, cognition and brain function with quantitative imaging evidence plays important role in elucidating both training and learning effects of college education that could advance further understanding of neurodevelopmental improvements during this crucial life-time period. The objectives of this chapter were to investigate the brain changes such as neural activity and myelin-related functional correlations as well as morphological/microstructural connectivity-based neuroplasticity enhancement during college training with longitudinal imaging and phenotypic data. Specifically, correlations between multiparametric imaging quantification including fALFF/ReHo/VMHC/GMD/FA and four aspects of EI including appraisal, monitoring/utilization of emotions and social ability as well as fluid intelligence and depression/anxiety scores at both cross-sectional and longitudinal scales were examined thoroughly with statistical analyses, comparisons and correlations.

2. Methods

2.1. Participants

This set of imaging and phenotypic data was downloaded after approval from the website managed at the NITRC database (www.nitrc.org). The multi-model MRI dataset including functional/structural/microstructural levels from a large cohort of adult lifespan sample was provided by the Southwest University at Chongqing City in China and College of Psychology (https://fcon_ 1000.projects.nitrc.org/indi/retro/sald.html), known as Southwest University Longitudinal Imaging Multimodal (SLIM) project. The main purpose of the SLIM project was to uncover the developmental trajectory of the human brain and understand the changes associated with aging, with the ultimate goal of discovering the causes of nervous system diseases related to aging. SLIM dataset of brain and phenotypic information with duration of three and a half years (acquired during years of 2011-2015) also included rich samples of behavior-related demographic, cognitive and emotional assessments [1, 3].

Participants were recruited from the Southwest University with the campus network and consisted of college students mainly. Each individual was screened to be healthy and no MRI contraindications, with exclusion criteria such as history of psychiatric disorder, cognitive disability or substance abuse. Demographic information of participants for available fMRI fALFF/ReHo/VMHC and structural VBM data are listed in Table 1 for initial time point 1 (TP1), intermediate follow-up time point 2 (TP2) and later time point (TP3). The mean age of 138 participants (83 women and 55 men) was 19.0 ± 0.6 years at initial TP1, and average follow-up of 1.1 ± 0.2 years at TP2 as well as 2.6 ± 0.3 years interval at TP3 from TP1. For the DTI, 564 participants with baseline age of 20.0 ± 1.0 years and two similar follow-up time points (1-3 years) were processed and compared.

Phenotypic Information	Scan Time 1	Scan Time 2	Scan Time 3
Age (years)	18.99 ± 0.62	20.22 ± 0.49	21.71 ± 0.41
Follow-up Time (years)	-	1.10 ± 0.23	2.59 ± 0.26
Intelligence Scale			
Appraisal of Emotion	36.31 ± 3.31	-	-
Monitor of Emotions	27.47 ± 2.25	-	-
Social Ability	21.06 ± 1.92	-	-
Utilization of Emotions	26.10 ± 2.29	-	-
Raven's CRT Score	62.08 ± 2.97	-	-
Neuropsychological Test Score			
Depression (BDI)	3.18 ± 1.27	8.23 ± 6.82	3.47 ± 1.96
State Anxiety (SAN)	28.00 ± 4.08	36.39 ± 9.82	21.94 ± 0.93
Trait Anxiety (TAN)	31.65 ± 5.11	39.59 ± 9.51	33.50 ± 4.87

Table 1. *Demographic information including age (19.0 ± 0.6 years at initial scan time 1), gender (83 women and 55 men with total of 138 participants and 60% women), mean follow-up time as well as phenotypic data including emotional intelligence (EI) scores of four aspects, combined Raven's Matrices test (CRT) score and neuropsychological measures including Beck's depression inventory (BDI), state anxiety (SAN) and trait anxiety (TAN) tests at three times*

Phenotypic data including emotional intelligence (EI) scores of four aspects, combined Raven's Matrices test (CRT) score and neuropsychological measures including Beck's depression inventory (BDI), state anxiety (SAN) and trait anxiety (TAN) tests at initial time point, and neuropsychological tests including anxiety/depression scores at two follow-up times (Table 1) were also collected for correlational analysis [37, 38].

2.2. Imaging Parameters and Data Processing

MRI experiments were performed using the 3T scanner with standardized imaging protocols. The 3D MPRAGE sequence was run with TR/TI/TE=1900/900/2.52 ms, flip angle=9°, matrix size=256 x 256 x 176, resolution=1 x 1x 1 mm³ for reference image used in resting-state (RS)-fMRI connectivity/conductivity maps, as well as for structural voxel-based morphometry (VBM) analysis. For the resting-state (RS)-fMRI data acquired under relaxing condition, a standard gradient-echo EPI sequence (TR/TE=2000/30 msec, flip angle=90°, number of volumes=242, spatial resolution=3.44 x 3.44 x 4 mm³) was utilized. DTI data was obtained with standard spin-echo EPI sequence (TR/TE=11000/98 msec, flip angle=90°, number of diffusion directions=30, three repetitions, b-value=1000 s/mm², spatial resolution=2 x 2 x 2 mm³).

The MRI and fMRI images were processed with the in-house developed scripts to derive the VMHC, VBM, ICA-DR, resting-state functional connectivity (RSFC) and fractional ALFF (fALFF) maps, as described in details in our previous chapters. Graph theory based small-worldness systematic analysis was computed to the functional connectivity of MRI (fcMRI) data with correlation matrix generated from 116 seeds-based RSFC, and comparisons between patients and controls were performed. In addition, regional homogeneity (ReHo) map was generated to reflect spatially local synchrony of spontaneous neuronal activities, after preprocessing the fMRI data such as motion correction and low-pass filtering [39, 40].

DTI data were first pre-processed with the Diffusion Toolkit toolbox (http://tractvis.org) to obtain the fractional anisotropy (FA) and three diffusivity metrics such as axial diffusivity (AD), radial diffusivity (RD) and mean diffusivity (MD) values in original B0 space. For the FA/RD/AD/MD quantification, the FSL tract-based spatial statistics (TBSS) toolbox steps 1–2 (i.e. preprocessing, brain mask extraction with FA>0.1 and normalization) were used for registration of all participants' FA into the FSL 1-mm white matter skeleton template. Statistical comparisons between each of three time points were performed to the voxel-wise whole brain and 20 tract-based FA/AD/RD/MD data. Both voxel-wise, regional functional and structural/micro-structural imaging quantification and longitudinal comparisons were also performed to examine any alterations during 3-4 year college training periods.

Correlational analysis between imaging quantifications and phenotypic data were performed with FSL toolbox including EI, aging effects and depression/anxiety scores. And statistical longitudinal comparisons as well as causal prediction of later neuropsychological measures with imaging data at earlier time points were also implemented for all the fMRI fALFF/ReHo/VMHC and structural VBM together with DTI metrics using the whole-brain voxel-wise analyses. Regional and tract-specific quantification of DTI metrics and correlations with phenotypic data were also performed together with the graph-theory based small-worldness efficiency analysis based on the multi-regional fMRI functional connectivity data at each time point [41, 42].

3. Results

Significant correlations between fALFF images and EI scores were illustrated in Figure 1 as A-C at three time points (TP) respectively (P<0.05). Increased EI associations in the visuospatial, medial and dorso-lateral frontal regions were observed from TP1 to TP2 and TP3; especially the positive correlations between the occipital/precuneal/cuneal/ cerebellar/motor neural activities and four EI sub-scores but negative correlations between orbitofrontal/medial/superior frontal (including ACC)/insular/ posterior cingulate neural fluctuation in low-frequency and EI metrics. Several regions including insula, basal ganglia, hypothalamus, thalamus, superior temporal region, posterior cingulate, cuneus, motor and supplementary motor areas also presented links between neural activity and four different aspects of

EI scores such as social ability and utilization at TP2 with small hypothalamus/insular neural activities relating to the EI at initial TP1. And initially, negative associations were only seen in scattered small regions of motor/supplementary motor and superior temporal areas between fALFF and EI metrics. As for trait associations, significant correlations between fALFF images and depression/anxiety traits scores (also including Raven's CRT metric) at three time points were displayed in Figure 2 with P<0.05 and A-C for TP1-TP3 respectively. Multiple regional associations were observed; for instance, positive correlation between orbitofrontal fALFF and BDI score as well as negative correlations between superior temporal fALFF and BDI score at TP1. Some similar regions as in EI association such as visuofrontal, motor/supplementary motor areas, thalamus and basal ganglia, posterior cingulate and temporoparietal regions also presented negative correlations with different aspects of the traits scores at three time points. Especially, correlational orbitofrontal and motor fALFF at TP1 and occipital fALFF with trait anxiety at TP3; insular/subcortical caudate fALFF with state anxiety at TP2, association between fALFF in the default mode nodes such as medial prefrontal and posterior cingulate as well as in the motor area with Raven's CRT score were observed. Figure 3 showed the fALFF prediction of trait scores including fALFF at TP1 and trait scores at TP2, fALFF at TP1 and trait scores at TP3, as well as fALFF at TP2 and trait scores at TP3 as in A-C respectively. Trait anxiety scores at later time TP2 and TP3 could be predicted by fALFF (neural activity) in the orbitofrontal, medial frontal and parietal/premotor areas at earlier TP1 and TP2 respectively with expected negative correlations. Superior temporal fALFF at earlier TP1 and TP2 predicted depression score at TP2 and TP3, and neural activity at TP1 in the motor/supplementary area also predicted depression score at TP2. In summary, neural activity in the regions of OFC and basal ganglia/thalamus predicted depression score longitudinally, and superior temporal fALFF predicted state and trait anxiety scores.

Significant correlations between ReHo images and EI scores at three time points (TP) respectively as A for TP1, B for TP2 and C for TP3 (P<0.05) were illustrated in Figure 4. Regions of orbitofrontal, ventral striatum, insula, hippocampus and superior frontal gyrus presented negative association between regional homogeneity (ReHo) and EI appraisal score at TP1, with more associated regions in the superior frontal regions and parahippocampus at TP3. Regions of scattered parietal clusters and premotor/motor areas also presented positive link between ReHo and EI monitoring and appraisal/social ability scores at TP2 primarily; on the other hand, ReHo of regions in the superior temporal cortex including insular and small dorsolateral frontal cluster correlated positively with the EI social ability score at TP2. Finally, ReHo at TP3 in the posterior cingulate, inferior temporal region including the fusiform together with anterior cingulate related positively to EI appraisal and utilization scores, and noticeably ReHo in the motor/premotor and superior temporal clusters correlated (also positive) with all four aspects of EI scores as well. Significant correlations between ReHo images and depression/anxiety traits scores (also including Raven's CRT metric) at three time points (TP) were displayed in Figure 5 A-C respectively (P<0.05). Regions of orbitofrontal and posterior cingulate presented positive associations with trait anxiety and depression scores at TP1, but with negative association found mainly in the cerebellum, superior temporal and insular regions. Orbito, medial and superior frontal regions presented positive link between ReHo and Raven's CRT score, but negative in the temporal cortex and cerebellum at TP1. At TP2, regions of scattered frontoparietal clusters and premotor/motor areas also presented negative link between ReHo and anxiety/depression trait scores. While insular/supplementary motor ReHo presented positive association with Raven's CRT score, but occipito-parietal ReHo correlated negatively with Raven's score at TP2 mostly. Finally at TP3, positive associations between ReHo values in the motor/premotor and small superior frontal/temporal regions with trait/state anxiety scores were exhibited. However, small clusters in the orbito-, medial and superior portions of frontal cortex showed negative associations between ReHo and trait anxiety score. ReHo in the superior temporal/insular/motor/supplementary motor areas showed positive correlation with Raven's CRT score, while negative in the frontal/ hippocampal/striatal clusters with Raven's score.

ReHo prediction of trait scores as ReHo metric at TP1 and trait scores at TP2, ReHo at TP1 and trait scores at TP3 as well as ReHo at TP2 and trait scores at TP3 were displayed in Figure 6 A-C. Longitudinal, ReHo prediction showed some similarity as cross-sectional correlations such as negative correlations between ReHo at TP1 in motor/parietal areas and TS metrics such as depression score at TP2, as well as between superior temporal/insular ReHo at TP1 and depression score at TP1. Also ReHo in precuneus, frontal pole and superior frontal region at TP1 related to depression scores at TP2 and TP3, while ReHo in the inferior parietal and superior temporo-occipital regions (left side mostly) predicted trait anxiety score at TP3. Finally, ReHo in the occipito-parietal region at TP2 predicted depression and state anxiety score at TP3.

Figure 7 presented longitudinal VMHC differences between TP2 and TP1 in the inferior temporal area, and between TP3 and TP1 in the posterior cingulate and inferior parietal regions. No other longitudinal changes of functional images such as fALFF/ ReHo/ICA-DR network connectivities were found comparing TP2 to TP1 or TP3 to TP2/TP1 time points. Correlation maps between VMHC and EI/TS scores were displayed in Figure 8 (P<0.05), for both cross-sectional and longitudinal predictions. At TP1, significant positive correlations between VMHC in the posterior cingulate/striatum regions and the depression scale existed, and posterior cingulate VMHC also linked to the state anxiety score. Additionally, occipital/precuneus/superior parietal VMHC values were associated with the trait anxiety score positively but negatively in the cerebellum and medial temporal lobe including parahippocampus. Also VMHC in large areas including the orbitofrontal, IFG, MPFC, superior temporal, posterior cingulate, occipital, supplementary motor regions and cerebellum were correlated positively with the Raven's CRT score. No significant correlations between VMHC and other EI scores were found at TP1 (Figure 8). At TP2, VMHC of small regions in the anterior cingulate, occipital/orbitofrontal and cerebellum correlated positively with the EI utilization score. Furthermore, VMHC in the cerebellum, temporal cortex including amygdala/hippocampus/parahippocampus and superior segment, sensorimotor area and occipital lobe showed consistently negative associations with the depression/anxiety scores at TP2. Moreover, cerebellar/occipital/orbitofrontal and superior frontal VMHC were linked to the Raven's CRT score negatively. Finally at TP3, parietal/temporal VMHC correlated with depression and anxiety scores negatively; on the other hand, orbitofrontal/striatal/supplementary motor VMHC related positively to the depression/trait anxiety scores but negatively to the Raven's CRT score. In addition, Figure 9 showed correlation maps between earlier VMHC and predicted later trait scores (P<0.05), and age correlations of three functional images at initial time point were also demonstrated. Interhemispheric correlations (Figure 9 A-C) in the temporal cortex including amygdala/hippocampus/parahippo-campus/superior temporal segments, occipital, posterior cingulate, somatomotor and supplementary motor areas, insular, striatum, basal ganglia and cerebellum at earlier time points (TP1 & TP2) could predict the depression/anxiety scores with negative correlations at later time points (TP2 & TP3). As for age correlations with functional quantifications, superior frontal/posterior occipital/striatal VMHC showed aging effect with positive association (Figure 9D). And ReHo values in the visual cortex including the lingual, cuneus and lateral occipital regions in addition to the small posterior cingulate/precuneus clusters also showed positive aging effect, while negative association found in the left superior temporal/insular region. Finally, occipital/ cerebellar fALFF linked positively to age, and right sensorimotor/motor fALFF related negatively to participant's age.

Significant correlations between VBM images for gray matter density and EI scores at three time points were demonstrated in Figure 10 (P<0.05). Strong positive correlations between gray matter density in the cerebellum, insular, orbitofrontal, fusiform, cuneus, posterior cingulate, medial prefrontal, subcortical caudate and putamen regions were observed with the EI scores of four domains including appraisal, monitoring, social ability and utilization at three time points. Gray matter density in regions of superior temporal, dorsolateral prefrontal, motor and supplementary motor areas presented negative association with EI scores in four sub-domains as well. Significant correlations between VBM images and trait scores at three time points were present in Figure 11 (P<0.05). Cortical temporal regions including hippocampus and parahippocampus, orbitofrontal and superior frontal, visual and sensorimotor areas demonstrated significant correlations with depression and trait/state anxiety scores mainly. Correlations at each time point and for different traits were spatially close with mild variations such as in the middle temporal, occipital and dorso-lateral frontal lobes. Interestingly, cuneal gray matter density correlated positively with Raven's CRT score but negatively with depression scale at all three time points, especially at TP1 and TP3. And finally, Figure 12 showed gray matter density prediction of trait scores (P<0.05). Similar regions such as the middle temporal cortex including amygdala, hippocampus, occipital, orbitofrontal, dorso-lateral prefrontal (DLPFC) and motor/supplementary motor areas as to the cross-sectional correlation results in Figure 11 were observed with less spatial spread; but more correlations were present in state anxiety prediction. Finally, no significant longitudinal changes of gray matter density at later time points (TP2 or TP3) compared to earlier time points (TP1 or TP2) were observed (P>0.05) with VBM results.

Figure 13 showed significant correlations between FA images and EI scores at three time points (P<0.05). Associations between EI appraisal score and FA in a few tracts including the thalamic radiation, splenium of corpus callosum, internal capsule, cingulum, superior longitudinal fasciculus and cortico-spinal tract were identified at both time points. No significant correlations between FA and EI at initial time point were found, and no longitudinal changes of FA values at later time points (TP2 & TP3) were observed either (P>0.05). Strong correlations between FA images and depression/anxiety traits scores (also including Raven's CRT score) at three time points were displayed in Figure 14 with P<0.05. Multiple regional associations were observed; for instance, positive correlation between fronto-occipital fasciculus and depression/state anxiety scores at TP1 but negative correlation at TP2. Positive correlations between cortico-spinal tract and depression score, as well as between cingulum/superior longitudinal fasciculus and state anxiety were also present at TP3. Moreover, stronger correlations between Raven's CRT score and tracts of cingulum, hippocampus, thalamic radiation, internal capsule, uncinate fasciculus were observed at TP3 compared to TP2 and TP1. Figure 15 showed FA prediction of trait scores (P<0.05), and the microstructural integrity of superior longitudinal fasciculus, cingulum, corpus callosum, inferior longitudinal fasciculus and cortico-spinal tracts at earlier time (TP1 and TP2) could predict anxiety/depression traits at later time (TP2 and TP3).

Significant correlations (P≤0.006) between DTI FA/AD/RD/MD tract-specific metrics and EI/TS cognitive scores at initial time point (TP1) were displayed in Figure 16. Diffusivities in the tracts of cingulum, inferior fronto-occipital fasciculus, inferior longitudinal fasciculus, uncinate fasciculus and minor forceps for memory, executive function and emotion regulation were tightly and negatively associated with the EI and TS phenotypic scores of emotion and intelligence. Figure 17 showed strong correlations (P≤0.05) between DTI FA/AD/RD/MD tract-specific metrics and EI/TS cognitive scores at time point 2 (TP2). Correlations at TP2 included similar tracts as to TP1 such as cingulum and superior longitudinal fasciculus (SLF), but with new cortico-spinal tract that linked to Raven's CRT score as well as major forceps that was related to the social ability. Furthermore, Figure 18 presented the significant correlations (P≤0.05) between DTI FA/AD/RD/MD tract-specific metrics and EI/TS cognitive scores at TP3. Diffusivities in the tracts of cingulum, superior longitudinal fasciculus, cortico-spinal tract, uncinate fasciculus and major forceps were related to the depression/trait anxiety/social ability and utilization of emotion scores at later TP3. Quantitative correlational results between tract-specific FA/diffusivity metrics and EI/traits are listed in Table 2 a-c for TP1-TP3 respectively.

Age correlation of DTI axial diffusivity (AD) and mean diffusivity (MD) were displayed in Figure 19A and gray matter density with VBM in Figure 19B (P<0.05) respectively. Negative associations were found between AD/MD with age in several brain tracts including inferior longitudinal fasciculus, cortico-spinal tract, thalamic radiation, inferior fronto-occipital fasciculus, cingulum and uncinate fasciculus. On the other hand, positive age correlation was found in the internal capsule with both limbs and cortico-spinal tract. Gray matter densities increased in the hippocampus, amygdala, ventral striatum, orbitofrontal, dorso-lateral frontal, inferior parietal and scattered occipital regions over time. Decreased gray matter density was also seen in the temporal, insular and cuneal regions with age.

Tract Name	Phenotypic Data	DTI	r	P
Inferior fronto-occipital fasciculus L	EI Appraisal of Emotions	RD	-0.166	0.0025
Inferior fronto-occipital fasciculus L	EI Appraisal of Emotions	MD	-0.161	0.0032
Inferior fronto-occipital fasciculus L	EI Social Ability	RD	-0.172	0.0017
Inferior fronto-occipital fasciculus L	EI Social Ability	MD	-0.172	0.0017
Uncinate fasciculus R	EI Social Ability	RD	-0.161	0.0032
Inferior fronto-occipital fasciculus L	EI Utilization of Emotions	RD	-0.154	0.0049
Uncinate fasciculus R	EI Utilization of Emotions	RD	-0.169	0.0020
Cingulum L	BDI	MD	-0.136	0.0043
Inferior fronto-occipital fasciculus L	BDI	MD	-0.132	0.0053
Superior longitudinal fasciculus L	BDI	MD	-0.131	0.0057
Superior longitudinal fasciculus L	SAN	RD	-0.140	0.0020
Forceps minor	SAN	RD	-0.140	0.0020
Inferior longitudinal fasciculus L	SAN	AD	-0.144	0.0014
Superior longitudinal fasciculus L	SAN	AD	-0.126	0.0053
Forceps minor	SAN	MD	-0.138	0.0023
Superior longitudinal fasciculus L	SAN	MD	-0.146	0.0013

Tract Name	Phenotypic Data	DTI	r	P
Superior longitudinal fasciculus L	TAN	AD	-0.118	0.0059
		MD	-0.123	0.0041

Table 2a. *Significant correlations (P<0.01) between phenotypic data (EI/trait scores) and DTI tracts with four metrics of DTI (FA, MD, AD and RD) and 20 tracts in at initial TP1. L=left, R=right. Expected correlation directions were highlighted in bold.*

Figure 20 identified significantly increased global efficiency and decreased local efficiency (both relative and absolute) at time point 3 (TP3) compared to time point 2 (TP2), with P<0.0001 for all four metrics. The small-worldness normalization factor was also decreased, indicating a more optimal and efficient brain network topology at later time point after college training. Enhanced results were found comparing TP3 to time point 1 (TP1) with both increased global absolute/relative and local absolute efficiencies (P<0.0001), while local relative efficiency and small-worldness factors were relatively close between two time points. Only global relative (Lamda) and local absolute (CCFS) efficiencies reached significance (P<0.05) comparing TP2 to TP1 with higher local but lower global efficiencies and increased small-worldness factor at TP2.

Tract Name	Phenotypic Data	DTI	r	P
Superior longitudinal fasciculus (tem) L	EI Appraisal of Emotions	FA	-0.158	0.0500
Cingulum R		AD	0.241	0.0025
Superior longitudinal fasciculus R			0.200	0.0128
Cingulum R		MD	0.220	0.0059
Cingulum (hippocampus) R			0.214	0.0076
Cingulum R	EI Monitor of Emotions	AD	0.229	0.0042
Superior longitudinal fasciculus R			0.188	0.0194
Cingulum R		MD	0.225	0.0048
Cingulum (hippocampus) R			0.202	0.0117
Forceps major	EI Social Ability	FA	-0.169	0.0358
Cingulum R		AD	0.223	0.0054
Superior longitudinal fasciculus R			0.226	0.0049
Cingulum (hippocampus) R		MD	0.159	0.0485
Cingulum R	EI Utilization of Emotions	AD	0.204	0.0110
Superior longitudinal fasciculus R			0.232	0.0039
Cortico-spinal tract L	**Raven's CRT**	**AD**	**-0.143**	**0.0489**
Cingulum R			0.172	0.0175

Table 2b. *Significant correlations (P<0.01) between phenotypic data and DTI tracts with four metrics of DTI (FA, MD, AD and RD) and 20 tracts in at TP2. L=left, R=right. tem=temporal part. Expected correlation directions were highlighted in bold.*

Tract Name	Phenotypic Data	DTI	r	P
Cingulum L	EI Social Ability	RD	-0.201	0.0217
Cortico-spinal tract L		AD	-0.174	0.0474
Cortico-spinal tract R		AD	-0.196	0.0256
Superior longitudinal fasciculus L		MD	-0.228	0.0091
		AD	-0.202	0.0212
Cingulum L	EI Utilization of Emotions	AD	-0.192	0.0289
Superior longitudinal fasciculus L		RD	-0.222	0.0110
		AD	-0.188	0.0322
Forceps major	BDI	RD	-0.214	0.0169
Uncinate fasciculus R		RD	-0.200	0.0259
Cingulum (hippocampus) L		AD	0.239	0.0074
Cingulum (hippocampus) R		AD	0.243	0.0065
Forceps major		MD	-0.213	0.0173
Uncinate fasciculus R		MD	-0.187	0.0373
Superior longitudinal fasciculus L	TAN	RD	-0.155	0.0201
		AD	-0.167	0.0122
Cingulum (hippocampus) R		MD	0.132	0.0480
Superior longitudinal fasciculus L		MD	-0.169	0.0113

Table 2c. *Significant correlations (P<0.01) between phenotypic data (EI/trait scores) and DTI tracts with four metrics of DTI (FA, MD, AD and RD) and 20 tracts in at TP3. L=left, R=right.*

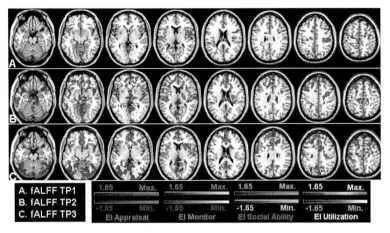

Figure 1. *Significant correlations between fALFF images and EI scores at three time points (TP) respectively as A for time point 1 (TP1), B for TP2 and C for TP3 (P<0.05). Increased EI associations in the visuospatial and medial and dorso-lateral frontal regions were observed from TP1 to TP2 and TP3; especially the positive correlations between the occipital/precuneal/cuneal/cerebellar/motor neural activities and four EI sub-scores (red/yellow/green/x-rain colors in C) but negative correlations between orbitofrontal/medial/superior frontal (including ACC)/ insular/posterior cingulate neural connectivity and EI metrics (violet, gold, cyan and x-hot colors in B and C). Several regions including insula, basal ganglia, hypothalamus, thalamus, superior temporal region, posterior cingulate, cuneus, motor and supplementary motor areas also presented positive links between neural activity and four different aspects of EI scores such as social ability and utilization at time point 2 (red/yellow/green/x-rain colors in B) with small hypothalamus/ insular neural activities relating to the EI at initial time point 1 (yellow/green/x-rain colors in A). Also initially, negative associations were only seen in scattered small regions of motor/supplementary motor and superior temporal areas between fALFF and EI metrics (violet, gold, cyan and x-hot colors in A).*

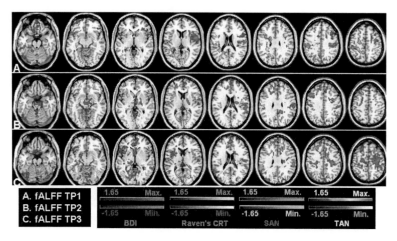

Figure 2. *Significant correlations between fALFF images and depression/anxiety traits scores (also including Raven's CRT metric) at three time points (TP) respectively as A for TP1, B for TP2 and C for TP3 (P<0.05). Multiple regional associations were observed; for instance, positive correlation between orbitofrontal fALFF and BDI score; negative correlations between superior temporal fALFF and BDI score at time point 1. Some similar regions as in Figure 1 including frontal, motor/supplementary motor areas, thalamus, basal ganglia, and temporoparietal regions also presented negative association with different aspects of the traits scores at three time points. Especially, correlational orbitofrontal and motor fALFF at TP1 and occipital fALFF with trait scores at TP3; insular/subcortical caudate fALFF with state anxiety at TP2 were observed. And positive association of Raven's CRT score and fALFF in the occipital, inferior and medial temporal, DLPFC, small caudate and thalamus were observed at three time points, in addition to the negative association between fALFF in the DMN such as medial prefrontal, superior frontal and posterior cingulate, parietal, premotor and motor areas.*

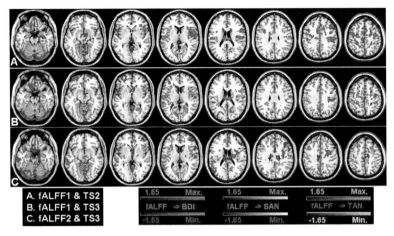

Figure 3. *fALFF prediction of trait scores as fALFF at time point 1 (fALFF1) and trait scores at time point 2 (TS2) in A; fALFF1 and TS3 in B as well as fALFF at time point 2 (fALFF2) and trait TS3 in C. Trait anxiety scores at time point 2 and 3 could be predicted by fALFF (neural activity) in the orbitofrontal, medial frontal and parietal/premotor areas at time point 1 (TP1) and 2 (TP2) respectively (green-cyan color). Superior temporal fALFF at time point1 and 2 predicted depression score at time point 2 and 3 (violet color), and neural activity at time point 1 in the motor/supplementary area linked to depression score at time point 2. Generally, neural activity in the regions of orbitofrontal and basal ganglia/thalamus predicted depression scores longitudinally, and superior temporal /motor/cuneus/inferior parietal fALFF predicted state anxiety score.*

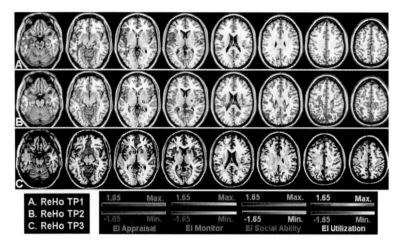

Figure 4. *Significant correlations between ReHo images and EI scores at three time points (TP) respectively as A for TP1, B for TP2 and C for TP3 (P<0.05). Regions of orbitofrontal and ventral striatum, insular, hippocampus and superior frontal gyrus presented negative association between regional homogeneity and EI appraisal score at time point 1 and more regions in the superior frontal regions and parahippocampus at time point 3 (violet color in A & C). Regions of scattered parietal clusters and premotor/motor areas also presented positive link between ReHo and EI monitoring and appraisal/social ability scores at time point 2 primarily (yellow, red, green and combined colors in B); and ReHo of regions in the superior temporal cortex including insular and small dorsolateral frontal cluster correlated positively with the EI social ability score (green color in B) at TP 2. Finally, at time point 3, ReHo in the posterior cingulate, inferior temporal region including the fusiform together with anterior cingulate related positively to EI appraisal and utilization scores (orange-red hot color in C), and noticeably motor/premotor and superior temporal clusters correlated positively with all four aspects of EI scores (mixed red, green, yellow and X-rain colors as X-rain color in C).*

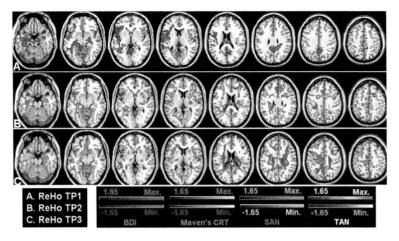

Figure 5. *Significant correlations between ReHo images and depression/anxiety traits scores (also including Raven's CRT metric) at three time points (TP) respectively as A for TP1, B for TP2 and C for TP3 (corrected, P<0.05). Regions of orbitofrontal and posterior cingulate presented positive associations with trait anxiety and depression scores at TP1 (red and x-rain color); however, negative correlations were found mainly in the cerebellum, superior temporal and insular regions (violet). Orbito, medial and superior frontal regions presented positive link between ReHo and Raven's CRT score (yellow), but negative in the temporal cortex and cerebellum at TP1 (gold). At TP2, Regions of scattered frontoparietal clusters and premotor/motor areas also presented negative link between ReHo and anxiety/depression scales (violet and x-hot colors). While insular/supplementary motor ReHo presented positive association with Raven's CRT score (yellow), but occipito-parietal ReHo correlated negatively with Raven's score at TP2 (gold). Finally at TP3, positive associations between ReHo values in the motor/premotor and small superior frontal/temporal regions with trait/state anxiety scores were exhibited (red, green and x-rain colors). However, small cluster in the frontal regions of the orbito, medial and superior portions showed negative associations between ReHo and trait anxiety score (x-hot color). ReHo in the superior temporal/insular/motor/supplementary motor areas showed positive correlation with Raven's CRT score (yellow), while negative in the frontal/hippo-campal/striatal clusters with Raven's score (gold).*

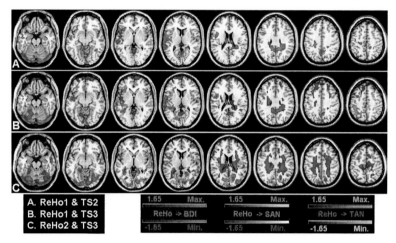

Figure 6. *ReHo prediction of trait scores as ReHo metric at time point 1 (ReHo1) and trait scores at time point 2 (TS2) for A together with ReHo at time point 1 (ReHo1) and trait scores at time point 3 (TS3) in B as well as ReHo at time point 2 (ReHo2) and trait scores at time point 3 in C. Longitudinal ReHo prediction showed some similarity as cross-sectional correlations such as correlations between ReHo1 in motor/parietal areas and TS metrics such as depression score at time point 2 (red color in C), as well as between superior temporal and insular ReHo1 and TS2/TS3 measuring depression and anxiety at time points 2 and 3 (negative violet, gold and cyan color in A and B). Also ReHo1 in precuneus, frontal pole and superior frontal region at time point 1 related to depression score at time points 2 and 3 (TS2 & TS3) (red color in A&B); and ReHo1 in the inferior parietal and temporo-occipital regions (left side mostly) correlated negatively with trait anxiety score at time point 3 (cyan color in B). Finally, ReHo2 in the cerebellar, occipito-parietal, superior temporal and insular and cuneus regions at time point 2 predicted depression and state anxiety scores at time point 3 (violet and gold colors, negative correlations in C).*

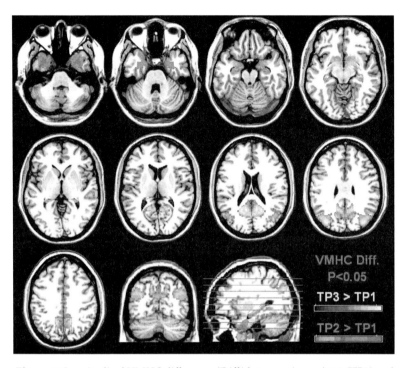

Figure 7. *Longitudinal VMHC differences (Diff.) between time point 2 (TP2) and time point 1 (TP1) in the inferior temporal area shown with violet color (P<0.05), and between time point 3 (TP3) and time point 1 (TP1) in the posterior cingulate and inferior parietal regions (yellow color).*

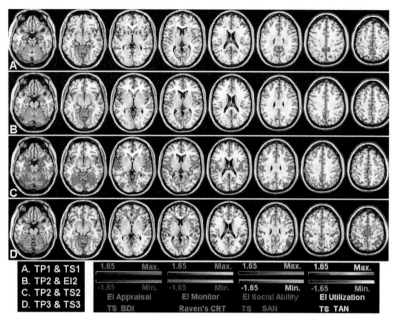

Figure 8. *Correlation maps between VMHC and EI/TS scores (P<0.05). A for correlation at TP1 between VMHC and traits score (TS1); B for VMHC at TP2 and EI score (EI2); C for VMHC images at time point 2 (TP2) and traits score (TS2); and D for VMHC at time point 3 (TP3) and traits score (TS3). At time point 1 (TP1) in A, significant correlations between VMHC in the posterior cingulate/striatum regions related positively to the depression scale (red color) and posterior cingulate VMHC also linked to the state anxiety score (green color). VMHC of large areas including the orbitofrontal, IFG, MPFC, superior temporal including parahippocampus, posterior cingulate, occipital, supplementary motor and cerebellum correlated to the Raven's CRT score (bright yellow color in A). No significant correlations between VMHC and other EI scores were found at TP1. At time point2, VMHC of small regions in the anterior cingulate, occipital/ orbitofrontal and cerebellum correlated with the EI utilization score (x-rain color in B). Also VMHC in the cerebellum, temporal cortex including amygdala/ hippocampus/parahippocampus and superior segment, sensorimotor area and occipital lobe showed consistently negative associations with the depression/ anxiety scores (violet, cyan and x-hot colors in C) at TP2. Moreover, cerebellar/occipital/orbitofrontal and superior frontal VMHC was linked to the Raven's CRT negatively (orange color). Finally at time point 3 in D, parietal/*

temporal/ cerebellar VMHC correlated with depression and anxiety scores negatively as well (violet, cyan and x-rain colors); on the other hand, orbitofrontal/striatal/supplementary motor/occipital VMHC related positively to the depression/trait anxiety scores (red and x-hot colors) but negatively to the Raven's CRT score (orange color).

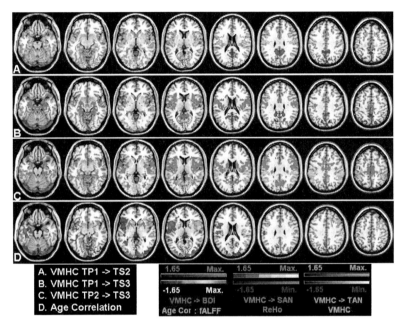

Figure 9. *Correlation maps between VMHC and trait scores (P<0.05). A for VMHC at time point 1 (TP1) and traits score at TP2 (TS2); B for VMHC at time point 1 (TP1) and traits score at TP3 (TS3); C for VMHC images at time point 2 (TP2) and traits score at TP3 (TS3). Age correlations of three functional images at initial time point 1 were demonstrated in D, including fALFF (red), ReHo (violet) and VMHC (green). Interhemispheric correlations (A-C) in the temporal cortex including amygdala/ hippocampus/parahippocampus/superior temporal segment, occipital, posterior cingulate, somatomotor and supplementary motor areas, insular, striatum, basal ganglia and cerebellum at earlier time points (TP1 & TP2) could predict the depression/anxiety scores at later time points (TP2 & TP3 with x-rain, violet and gold colors). The prediction of VMHC for trait scores increased longitudinally from TP1 to TP2, and more tightly linked with larger spatial spread at later time. Small clusters in the posterior cingulate/cuneus and lateral occipital*

regions presented positive correlations between VMHC and depression/state anxiety scale (red and green colors in A&B). D: As for age correlations with functional quantifications, posterior occipital/striatal VMHC showed aging effects (green color) with positive association. And ReHo values in the visual cortex including the lingual, cuneus and lateral occipital regions together with small clusters of posterior cingulate/precuneus also showed positive aging effect (orange color) but negative association in the left superior temporal/insular region. Finally, occipital/cerebellar fALFF linked positively to age (red color), while right sensorimotor/motor fALFF was negatively correlated with participant's age (x-rain color).

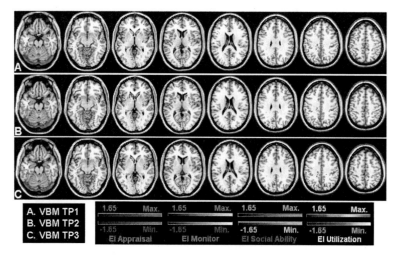

Figure 10. *Significant correlations between VBM images for gray matter density and EI scores at three time points (TP) respectively as A for TP1, B for TP2 and C for TP3 (P<0.05). Significant positive correlations between gray matter density in the cerebellum, insular, orbitofrontal, fusiform, cuneus, posterior cingulate, medial prefrontal, subcortical caudate and putamen regions were observed with the EI scores of four domains including appraisal, monitoring, social ability and utilization at three time points (red, yellow, green and mixed x-hot color). Gray matter density in regions of superior temporal, dorsolateral prefrontal, motor and supplementary motor areas presented negative association with EI scores in four sub-domains as well (violet, gold, cyan and mixed hot colors).*

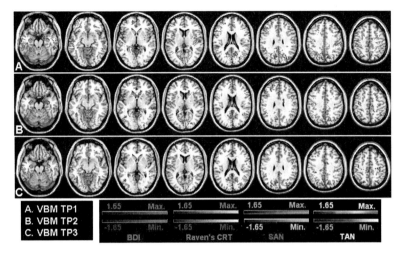

A. VBM TP1				
B. VBM TP2				
C. VBM TP3	BDI	Raven's CRT	SAN	TAN

Figure 11. *Significant correlations between gray matter density (GBM) images from VBM algorithm and trait scores at three time points (TP) respectively as A for TP1, B for TP2 and C for TP3 (P<0.05). Cortical temporal including hippocampus and parahippocampus, orbitofrontal and superior frontal, visual and sensorimotor areas demonstrated significant correlations with depression and trait/state anxiety scores mainly. Correlations at each time point and for different traits were spatially close with mild variations such as in the middle temporal, occipital and dorso-lateral frontal lobes. Interestingly, cuneal gray matter density correlated positively with Raven's CRT score (yellow color) but negatively with depression scale (violet) at all three time points, especially TP1 and TP3.*

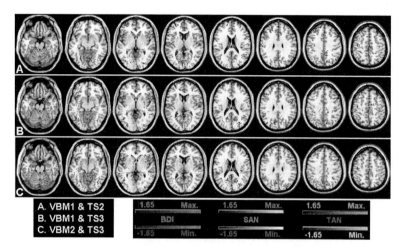

Figure 12. *Gray matter density prediction of trait scores: significant longitudinal correlations between VBM metric at time point 1 (VBM1) and trait scores at time point 2 (TS2) for A; VBM1 and trait scores at time point 3 (TS3) in B as well as VBM at time point 2 (VBM2) and TS3 in C (P<0.05). Similar to the cross-sectional correlation in Figure 11, regions in the middle temporal including amygdala, hippocampus, occipital, orbitofrontal, dorso-lateral prefrontal (DLPFC) and motor/supplementary motor areas exhibited GMD prediction for traits, with less spatial spread and more correlations present in state anxiety prediction (yellow and gold colors).*

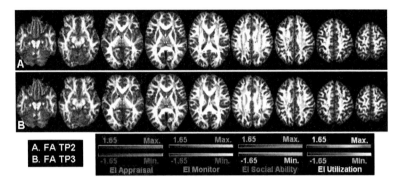

Figure 13. *Significant correlations between FA images and EI scores at three time points (TP) as A for TP2 and B for TP3 (P<0.05). No significant correlations between FA and EI at initial time point 1 (TP1) were found, and no longitudinal changes of FA at later time points were observed either (P>0.05). Associations between EI appraisal score/social ability/utilization and FA in a few tracts including the thalamic radiation, splenium of corpus callosum, internal capsule, cingulum, superior longitudinal fasciculus and cortico-spinal tract were identified at both later time points of TP2 and TP3.*

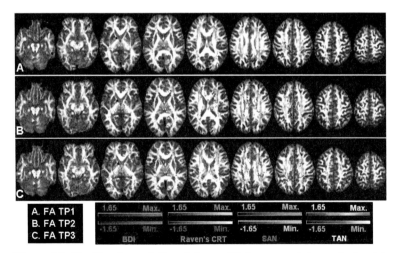

Figure 14. *Significant correlations between FA images and depression/anxiety traits scores (also including Raven's CRT metric) at three time points (TP) respectively as A for TP1, B for TP2 and C for TP3 (P<0.05) respectively. Multiple regional associations were observed; for instance, positive correlation between*

fronto-occipital tracts and BDI state anxiety score at time point 1; but negative correlations at time point 2. Positive correlations between cortico-spinal tract and depression score, as well as between cingulum/superior longitudinal fasciculus and state anxiety with interleaved positive and negative associations along the tracts were also present at time point 3. Stronger correlations between Raven's CRT score and tracts of cingulum, hippocampus, thalamic radiation, internal capsule, uncinate fasciculus were observed at TP3 compared to TP2 and TP1.

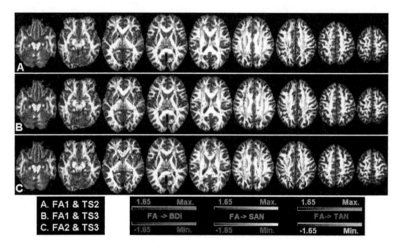

Figure 15. *FA prediction of trait scores: significant longitudinal correlations between FA at time point 1 (FA1) and trait scores at time point 2 (TS2) for A; FA1 and trait scores at time point 3 (TS3) in B as well as FA at time point 2 (FA2) and TS3 in C (P<0.05). Integrity of superior longitudinal fasciculus, cingulum, corpus callosum, inferior longitudinal fasciculus and cortico-spinal tracts at earlier time (TP1 and TP2) could predict anxiety/depression traits at later time (TP2 and TP3).*

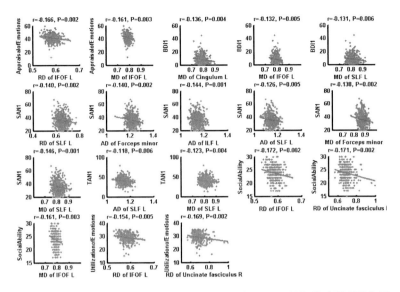

Figure 16. *Significant correlations (P≤0.006) between DTI FA/AD/RD/MD tract-specific metrics and EI/TS cognitive scores at initial time point 1 (TP1). IFOF=Inferior fronto-occipital fasciculus; SLF=Superior longitudinal fasciculus; ILF=Inferior longitudinal fasciculus; L=Left, R=Right. Diffusivities in the tracts of cingulum, inferior fronto-occipital fasciculus, inferior longitudinal fasciculus, uncinate fasciculus and minor forceps for memory, executive function and emotion were strongly and negatively associated with the EI such as social ability and appraisal/utilization of emotions, as well as TS phenotypic scores of emotion and intelligence.*

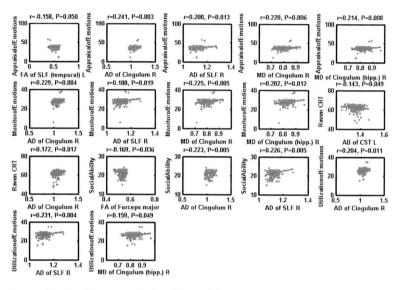

Figure 17. *Significant correlations (P≤0.05) between DTI FA/AD/RD/MD tract-specific metrics and EI/TS cognitive scores at middle time point 2 (TP2). SLF=Superior longitudinal fasciculus; CST=cortico-spinal tract; hippo.=hippocampus; L=Left, R=Right. Correlations at TP2 including similar tracts as to initial TP1 such as between cingulum and SLF, as well as new links between cortico-spinal tract and Raven's CRT score, between major forceps and the EI social ability score.*

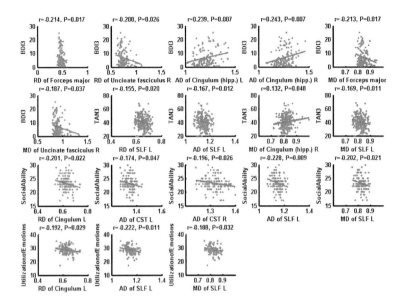

Figure 18. *Significant correlations (P≤0.05) between DTI FA/AD/RD/MD tract-specific metrics and EI/TS cognitive scores at later time point 3 (TP3). SLF=Superior longitudinal fasciculus; CST=cortico-spinal tract; hippo.=hippocampus; L=Left, R=Right. Diffusivities in the tracts of cingulum, superior longitudinal fasciculus, cortico-spinal tract, uncinate fasciculus and major forceps were related to the depression/trait anxiety/social ability and utilization of emotion scores at later TP3.*

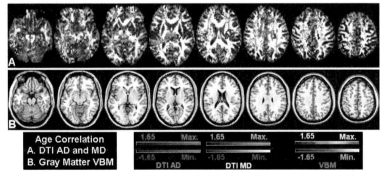

Figure 19. *Age correlation of DTI axial diffusivity (AD) and mean diffusivity (MD) in A and gray matter density with VBM in B (P<0.05). Negative associations were present between axial and mean diffusivities (AD and MD) and*

age in several brain tracts including inferior longitudinal fasciculus, cortico-spinal tract, thalamic radiation, inferior fronto-occipital fasciculus, cingulum and uncinate fasciculus (violet and yellow colors in A). On the other hand, positive age correlations were found in small clusters in the internal capsule with both limbs and cortico-spinal tract (red and green colors in A). Gray matter density increased in the hippocampus, amygdala, ventral striatum, orbitofrontal, dorso-lateral frontal, inferior parietal and scattered occipital regions (green and x-rain colors in B) with slightly elderly age. Decreased gray matter densities were also seen in the temporal, insular and cuneus regions in older individuals as negative correlation shown in x-hot color.

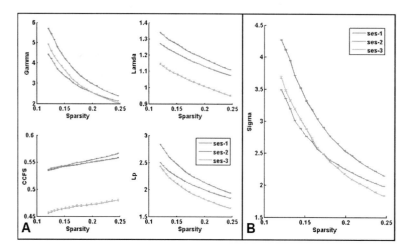

Figure 20. *Significantly increased global efficiency and decreased local efficiency (both relative and absolute) at time point 3 (TP3) compared to time point 2 (TP2), with P<0.0001 for all four metrics in A and decreased small-worldness normalization factor in B. Enhanced results were found comparing TP3 to time point 1 (TP1) with both increased global absolute/relative and local absolute efficiencies (P<0.0001), while local relative efficiency and small-worldness factors were relatively close between two time points. Only global relative (Lamda) and local absolute (CCFS) efficiencies reached significance (P<0.05) comparing TP2 to TP1 with higher local but lower global efficiencies and increased small-worldness factor at TP2.*

4. Discussion

4.1. Summary of Results

For the fALFF correlational results, several regions presented significantly positive correlations between fALFF neural activities and four aspects of EI scores including insula, hypothalamus, cuneus and motor areas at all three time points. Longitudinally, increased associations between fALFF and EI scores were observed in the visuospatial regions, medial and dorso-lateral prefrontal portions. Negative associations were also present in a few clusters such as the orbitofrontal cortex, posterior cingulate and superior frontal regions. For trait association, fALFF neural activities in some similar regions such as frontal, motor/supplementary motor areas, thalamus, basal ganglia and temporoparietal regions also revealed negative associations with different aspects of the traits scores at three time points. A few other regions including the orbitofrontal and occipital fALFF correlated positively with trait anxiety and depression scores. And fALFF in the occipital, inferior and medial temporal, DLPFC, small caudate and thalamus presented positive association with Raven's CRT score. However, some negative associations in the DMN, premotor and motor areas also existed, possibly due to the conventional compensation role of these negative associated regions. In terms of prediction, fALFF (neural activity) in the orbitofrontal, medial frontal and parietal/premotor areas at earlier TP1 and TP2 related to trait anxiety scores at later time of TP2 and TP3, while superior temporal /motor/cuneus/ inferior parietal fALFF predicted state anxiety score. Furthermore, neural activity values in the regions of orbitofrontal and basal ganglia/thalamus at earlier time points were positively associated with depression scores at later time, and superior temporal/ motor/supplementary motor fALFF predicted depression with negative association.

For the ReHo associations, EI scores including all four aspects were positively associated with regional homogeneity in the parietal/superior temporal cluster and premotor/motor areas during especially later time point 3 (TP3) and earlier TP2. While further regions of posterior cingulate, inferior temporal cortex including the fusiform together with anterior cingulate related positively to EI appraisal and utilization scores at TP3. Regarding the trait association, negative association was found mainly in the superior frontal and insular region. Regions of scattered frontoparietal clusters and premotor/motor areas also presented negative link between ReHo and anxiety/depression scores at TP2. During all the three time points, Raven's CRT score was positively associated with ReHo values in the orbitofrontal and superior frontal, insular, superior temporal and motor/supplementary motor areas. For the trait prediction, similar correlation results as to the cross-sectional findings were found, including negative correlations between earlier ReHo values in motor/parietal/temporo-occipital regions and later trait metrics such as depression and anxiety scores.

For the VMHC, significant longitudinal increments in the inferior temporal area at TP2 compared to TP1 were observed, together with the posterior cingulate and inferior parietal regions comparing TP3 to TP1 time points. Also VMHC correlated negatively with the trait scores in the cerebellum and medial temporal lobe at TP1, while parietal/temporal VMHC correlated with depression and anxiety scores at TP3. Moreover, VMHC of large areas including the orbitofrontal, IFG, MPFC, superior temporal including parahippocampus, posterior cingulate, occipital, supplementary motor and cerebellum correlated to the Raven's CRT score at TP1. At TP2, VMHC values in the cerebellum, temporal cortex including hippocampus/parahippocampus and superior segment, sensorimotor area and occipital lobe showed consistently negative associations with the depression/anxiety scores. For the prediction,

VMHC in the temporal cortex including hippocampus/parahippo-campus/ superior temporal segment, occipital, posterior cingulate, somatomotor and supplementary motor areas, insular, striatum, basal ganglia and cerebellum at earlier time point had been revealed to predict trait scores at later time. The prediction of VMHC for trait scores increased longitudinally from TP1 to TP2, and more tightly linked with larger spatial spread at later time as well as enhanced negative associations for depression and state anxiety especially. VMHC only correlated with EI scores at TP2, including interhemispheric correlations of small regions in the anterior cingulate, occipital/orbitofrontal and cerebellum association with the EI utilization score. As for aging effects, ReHo values in the left superior temporal/insular region and fALFF values in the right sensorimotor/motor area showed negative correlation, while VMHC/fALFF/ReHo in large areas of occipital lobe showed positive correlation with participant's age.

On the other hand, structural gray matter density and white matter fractional anisotropy showed fewer correlations with the EI and traits scores compared to functional imaging metrics. Particularly, significantly positive correlations between gray matter density in small clusters of the cerebellum, insular, orbitofrontal, fusiform, cuneus, posterior cingulate, medial prefrontal, subcortical caudate and putamen regions were observed with the EI scores of four domains at three time points. While cortical temporal regions including hippocampus and parahippocampus, orbitofrontal and superior frontal, visual and sensorimotor areas demonstrated significant correlations and predictions with depression and trait/state anxiety scores mainly. Associations between EI appraisal score and FA in a few tracts including the thalamic radiation, splenium of corpus callosum, internal capsule, cingulum, superior longitudinal fasciculus and cortico-spinal tract were identified at later time points TP2 and TP3. Correlations between cortico-spinal tract and depression score, as well as between cingulum/superior longitudinal fasciculus and state anxiety with interleaved positive and negative associations were discovered. Finally, diffusivities metrics including AD and RD from several tracts including cingulum, superior longitudinal fasciculus, cortico-spinal tract, uncinate fasciculus and major forceps showed expected correlations with EI and traits scores. Age-related gray matter density decreases were also observed in small temporal, insular and cuneus regions in individuals at initial time point, and axial/mean diffusivity values increased with age in small clusters in the internal capsule with both limbs and cortico-spinal tract. Also axial and mean diffusivities (AD and MD) were negatively associated with age in several brain tracts including inferior longitudinal fasciculus, cortico-spinal tract, thalamic radiation, inferior fronto-occipital fasciculus, cingulum and uncinate fasciculus. And significantly increased global efficiency and decreased local efficiency at later TP3 compared to TP2 and TP1 were identified, indicating a more optimal and efficient brain network topology at later time point after college training.

Given the population of this study that was college students with follow-up times of one-year and three-year educational experience, the quantitative results in this chapter were most likely reflecting the training and learning benefits for important qualify of life improvements in several aspects including knowledge of arts and science, characteristics, creativity, emotional regulation, vision, intelligence and social abilities. Further after-college follow-ups and correlation with other phenotypic profile such as creativity and quality-of-life index will be explored in the future studies.

4.2. Relating to Other Published Works

EI had been found to modulate the neural mechanism underlying the cognitive control tasks, and could be predicted by the working memory updating for emotional stimuli in females [43, 44]. The FPN together with the anterior insular and MPFC were activated for sustained emotional feelings in participants, aside from the regions for emotional images and words [45]. In addition, the cerebellar functional network contributed to all intrinsic networks via multiple, interdigitated (i.e., internal modeled) and spatially ordered mode to monitor and synchronize main cortical networks of cognition and emotion [46]. Moreover, performance-based ability EI seemed to have higher emotional processing abilities, and was validated in another study for specific performance-based working memory capacity tests [47, 48]. Arts, especially performance arts such as music, painting and dancing could stimulate brain and gain neuroplasticity, posing positive therapeutic effects to brain neurological injuries [49].

A common model of cognition (CMC) had been proposed based on the human connectome data analysis with a shared architectural artificial intelligence principle that subserved brain function across multiple cognitive domains [50]. Simultaneous activations of several large-scale neuronal networks such as DMN, CEN and SN, all consisting of frontal and parietal regions, were the characteristics of highly creative and innovative individuals [51]. Interactions among several neural systems of the creative cognition and drive as well as associated neuromodulatory systems could be further integrated to elucidate the creativity, motivation, mood and states that shaped human mind and idea production process [52]. For instance, it had been reported that DMN and CEN were cooperated dynamically to support complex cognitive processes including goal-directed self-reference [53]. Increased functional connectivity between bilateral inferior parietal cortex and dorsolateral prefrontal cortex was found in high-creativity group, suggesting greater cooperation between cognitive control and imaginative processes in brain [54]. Further longitudinal analysis revealed that slower rate of gray matter atrophy in the left frontoparietal and right frontotemporal clusters enhanced creativity, and right DLPFC was the most robust predictor of future creativity ability in young adults over follow-up interval of three years [55]. Also age-specific changes in productivity-related functional connectivity network were present in several typical networks such as DMN, CEN, FPN, SN, VN and cerebellum, with more spatial spread in younger compared to older adults [56].

4.3. Conclusion

In this chapter, we had investigated neural correlates of emotional intelligence and depression/anxiety traits at both cross-sectional and two longitudinal time points for a representative college-based population. For instance, fALFF/ReHo/VMHC in inferior parietal, motor/premotor and frontal regions including orbitofrontal and superior frontal segments as well as temporal cortex such as hippocampus were correlated with intelligence scores and trait metrics. In line with the results presented in previous two chapters, these regions showed improvements of neural activity, synchrony and integration, myelin-related conductivity, morphological and microstructural connectivity for better performance during skills training and knowledge accumulation. Also significantly increased global efficiency and decreased local efficiency at later time point TP3 compared to earlier time points TP2 and TP1 were identified, indicating a more optimal, ordered and efficient brain network topology at later time point after college training. Reviews of emotional and general intelligence as well as anxiety/depression neuroimaging findings together with related topics such as cortical mapping and CMC for arts/science and creativity provided further validation and confirmation. Consistent with reported findings, our integrative functional and structural results indicated expected and quantitative brain neuroplasticity enhancement during 3-4 year college education and learning periods that might gain long-term wisdom/creativity and could help protect against disease challenge.

References

[1] Chen Q, Beaty RE, Wei D, Yang J, Sun J, Liu W, Yang W, Zhang Q, Qiu J. Longitudinal Alterations of Frontoparietal and Frontotemporal Networks Predict Future Creative Cognitive Ability. Cereb Cortex. 2018 Jan 1;28(1):103-115. doi: 10.1093/cercor/bhw353. PMID: 29253252.

[2] Mayer JD, Salovey P, Caruso DR, Sitarenios G. Emotional intelligence as a standard intelligence. Emotion. 2001 Sep;1(3):232-42. PMID: 12934682.

[3] He L, Mao Y, Sun J, Zhuang K, Zhu X, Qiu J, Chen X. Examining Brain Structures Associated With Emotional Intelligence and the Mediated Effect on Trait Creativity in Young Adults. Front Psychol. 2018 Jun 15;9:925. doi: 10.3389/fpsyg.2018.00925. PMID: 29962984; PMCID: PMC6014059.

[4] Hakanen EA. Relation of emotional intelligence to emotional recognition and mood management. Psychol Rep. 2004 Jun;94(3 Pt 1):1097-103. doi: 10.2466/pr0.94.3.1097-1103. PMID: 15217076.

[5] Satary Dizaji A, Vieira BH, Khodaei MR, Ashrafi M, Parham E, Hosseinzadeh GA, Salmon CEG, Soltanianzadeh H. Linking Brain Biology to Intellectual Endowment: A Review on the Associations of Human Intelligence With Neuroimaging Data. Basic Clin Neurosci. 2021 Jan-Feb;12(1):1-28. doi: 10.32598/bcn.12.1.574.1. Epub 2021 Jan 1. PMID: 33995924; PMCID: PMC8114859.

[6] Karle KN, Ethofer T, Jacob H, Brück C, Erb M, Lotze M, Nizielski S, Schütz A, Wildgruber D, Kreifelts B. Neurobiological correlates of emotional intelligence in voice and face perception networks. Soc Cogn Affect Neurosci. 2018 Feb 1;13(2):233-244. doi: 10.1093/scan/nsy001. PMID: 29365199; PMCID: PMC5827352.

[7] Tan Y, Zhang Q, Li W, Wei D, Qiao L, Qiu J, Hitchman G, Liu Y. The correlation between emotional intelligence and gray matter volume in university students. Brain Cogn. 2014 Nov;91:100-7. doi: 10.1016/j.bandc.2014.08.007. Epub 2014 Oct 6. PMID: 25282329.

[8] Shi B, Cao X, Chen Q, Zhuang K, Qiu J. Different brain structures associated with artistic and scientific creativity: a voxel-based morphometry study. Sci Rep. 2017 Feb 21;7:42911. doi: 10.1038/srep42911. PMID: 28220826; PMCID: PMC5318918.

[9] Zhu W, Chen Q, Tang C, Cao G, Hou Y, Qiu J. Brain structure links everyday creativity to creative achievement. Brain Cogn. 2016 Mar;103:70-6. doi: 10.1016/j.bandc.2015.09.008. PMID: 26855062.

[10] Xurui T, Yaxu Y, Qiangqiang L, Yu M, Bin Z, Xueming B. Mechanisms of Creativity Differences Between Art and Non-art Majors: A Voxel-Based Morphometry Study. Front Psychol. 2018 Dec 11;9:2319. doi: 10.3389/fpsyg.2018.02319. PMID: 30618898; PMCID: PMC6301215.

[11] Zhu F, Zhang Q, Qiu J. Relating inter-individual differences in verbal creative thinking to cerebral structures: an optimal voxel-based morphometry study. PLoS One. 2013 Nov 5;8(11):e79272. doi: 10.1371/journal.pone.0079272. PMID: 24223921; PMCID: PMC3818430.

[12] Yang W, Liu P, Wei D, Li W, Hitchman G, Li X, Qiu J, Zhang Q. Females and males rely on different cortical regions in Raven's Matrices reasoning capacity: evidence from a voxel-based morpho-metry study. PLoS One. 2014 Mar 25;9(3):e93104. doi: 10.1371/journal.pone.0093104. PMID: 24667298; PMCID: PMC3965537.

[13] Yang J, Tian X, Wei D, Liu H, Zhang Q, Wang K, Chen Q, Qiu J. Macro and micro structures in the dorsal anterior cingulate cortex contribute to individual differences in self-monitoring. Brain Imaging Behav. 2016 Jun;10(2):477-85. doi: 10.1007/s11682-015-9398-0. PMID: 25958159.

[14] Javadi AH, Schmidt DH, Smolka MN. Differential representation of feedback and decision in adolescents and adults. Neuropsychologia. 2014 Apr;56(100):280-8. doi: 10.1016/j.neuropsychologia.2014.01. 021. Epub 2014 Feb 7. PMID: 24513024; PMCID: PMC3991323.

[15] Zhuang Q, Xu L, Zhou F, Yao S, Zheng X, Zhou X, Li J, Xu X, Fu M, Li K, Vatansever D, Kendrick KM, Becker B. Segregating domain-general from emotional context-specific inhibitory control systems - ventral striatum and orbitofrontal cortex serve as emotion-cognition integration hubs. Neuroimage. 2021 Sep;238:118269. doi: 10.1016/j.neuroimage.2021.118269. Epub 2021 Jun 15. PMID: 34139360.

[16] Bajaj S, Killgore WDS. Association between emotional intelligence and effective brain connectome: A large-scale spectral DCM study. Neuroimage. 2021 Apr 1;229:117750. doi: 10.1016/j.neuroimage. 2021.117750. Epub 2021 Jan 14. PMID: 33454407.

[17] Ling G, Lee I, Guimond S, Lutz O, Tandon N, Nawaz U, Öngür D, Eack S, E Lewandowski K, Keshavan M, Brady R Jr. Individual variation in brain network topology is linked to emotional intelligence. Neuroimage. 2019 Apr 1;189:214-223. doi: 10.1016/j.neuroimage.2019.01.013. Epub 2019 Jan 8. PMID: 30630078; PMCID: PMC6800254.

[18] Sawaya H, Johnson K, Schmidt M, Arana A, Chahine G, Atoui M, Pincus D, George MS, Panksepp J, Nahas Z. Resting-state functional connectivity of antero-medial prefrontal cortex sub-regions in major depression and relationship to emotional intelligence. Int J Neuropsychopharmacol. 2015 Mar 5;18(6):pyu112. doi: 10.1093/ijnp/pyu112. PMID: 25744282; PMCID: PMC4438550.

[19] Cun L, Wang Y, Zhang S, Wei D, Qiu J. The contribution of regional gray/white matter volume in preclinical depression assessed by the Automatic Thoughts Questionnaire: a voxel-based morphometry study. Neuroreport. 2014 Sep 10;25(13):1030-7. doi: 10.1097/WNR.0000000000000222. PMID: 24999908.

[20] Du X, Luo W, Shen Y, Wei D, Xie P, Zhang J, Zhang Q, Qiu J. Brain structure associated with automatic thoughts predicted depression symptoms in healthy individuals. Psychiatry Res. 2015 Jun 30;232(3):257-63. doi: 10.1016/j.pscychresns. 2015.03.002. Epub 2015 Mar 14. PMID: 25914142.

[21] Li W, Yang J, Zhang Q, Li G, Qiu J. The Association between Resting Functional Connectivity and Visual Creativity. Sci Rep. 2016 May 3;6:25395. doi: 10.1038/srep25395. PMID: 27138732; PMCID: PMC4853707.

[22] Wei D, Yang J, Li W, Wang K, Zhang Q, Qiu J. Increased resting functional connectivity of the medial prefrontal cortex in creativity by means of cognitive stimulation. Cortex. 2014 Feb;51:92-102. doi: 10.1016/j.cortex.2013.09.004. Epub 2013 Oct 2. PMID: 24188648.

[23] Pisner DA, Smith R, Alkozei A, Klimova A, Killgore WD. Highways of the emotional intellect: white matter microstructural correlates of an ability-based measure of emotional intelligence. Soc Neurosci. 2017 Jun;12(3):253-267. doi: 10.1080/17470919.2016.1176600. Epub 2016 May 9. PMID: 27072165.

[24] Chou KH, Cheng Y, Chen IY, Lin CP, Chu WC. Sex-linked white matter microstructure of the social and analytic brain. Neuroimage.

2011   Jan   1;54(1):725-33.   doi: 10.1016/j.neuroimage.2010.07.010.
Epub 2010 Jul 12. PMID: 20633662.

[25] Wertz CJ, Chohan MO, Ramey SJ, Flores RA, Jung RE. White matter
correlates of creative cognition in a normal cohort. Neuroimage. 2020
Mar;208:116293. doi: 10.1016/j.neuroimage.2019.116293. Epub 2019
Nov 27. PMID: 31785421.

[26] Blain SD, Grazioplene RG, Ma Y, DeYoung CG. Toward a Neural
Model   of   the   Openness-Psychoticism   Dimension: Functional
Connectivity in the Default and Frontoparietal Control Networks.
Schizophr Bull. 2020 Apr 10;46(3):540-551. doi: 10.1093/schbul/sbz103.
PMID: 31603227; PMCID: PMC7147581.

[27] Zhou J, Lo OY, Halko MA, Harrison R, Lipsitz LA, Manor B. The
functional implications and modifiability of resting-state brain
network complexity in older adults. Neurosci Lett. 2020 Feb
16;720:134775. doi: 10.1016/j.neulet.2020.134775. Epub 2020 Jan 20.
PMID: 31972253; PMCID: PMC7069223.

[28] Che X, Zhang Q, Zhao J, Wei D, Li B, Guo Y, Qiu J, Liu Y. Synchronous
activation within the default mode network correlates with perceived
social support. Neuropsychologia. 2014 Oct;63:26-33. doi: 10.1016/
j.neuropsychologia.2014.07.035. Epub 2014 Aug 8. PMID: 25111033.

[29] Tian X, Wei D, Du X, Wang K, Yang J, Liu W, Meng J, Liu H, Liu G,
Qiu J. Assessment of trait anxiety and prediction of changes in state
anxiety   using   functional   brain   imaging: A   test-retest   study.
Neuroimage.   2016   Jun;133:408-416.   doi: 10.1016/j.neuroimage.
2016.03.024. Epub 2016 Mar 19. PMID: 27001499.

[30] Steffens DC, Wang L, Manning KJ, Pearlson GD. Negative Affectivity,
Aging, and Depression: Results From the Neurobiology of Late-Life
Depression   (NBOLD)   Study.   Am   J   Geriatr   Psychiatry.   2017
Oct;25(10):1135-1149.   doi: 10.1016/j.jagp.2017.03.017.   Epub   2017
Apr 3. PMID: 28457805; PMCID: PMC5600659.

[31] Zilverstand A, Parvaz MA, Goldstein RZ. Neuroimaging cognitive
reappraisal in clinical populations to define neural targets for
enhancing emotion regulation. A systematic review. Neuroimage.
2017   May   1;151:105-116.   doi: 10.1016/j.neuroimage.2016.06.009.
Epub 2016 Jun 8. PMID: 27288319; PMCID: PMC5145785.

[32] Bang H, Zhou Y. The function of wisdom dimensions in ego-identity
development among Chinese university students. Int J Psychol. 2014

Dec;49(6):434-45. doi: 10.1002/ijop.12065. Epub 2014 Apr 4. PMID: 25355666.

[33] Extremera N, Fernández-Berrocal P, Salovey P. Spanish version of the Mayer-Salovey-Caruso Emotional Intelligence Test (MSCEIT). Version 2.0: reliabilities, age and gender differences. Psicothema. 2006;18 Suppl:42-8. PMID: 17295956.

[34] Lopes PN, Brackett MA, Nezlek JB, Schütz A, Sellin I, Salovey P. Emotional intelligence and social interaction. Pers Soc Psychol Bull. 2004 Aug;30(8):1018-34. doi: 10.1177/0146167204264762. PMID: 15257786.

[35] Navarro-Bravo B, Latorre JM, Jiménez A, Cabello R, Fernández-Berrocal P. Ability emotional intelligence in young people and older adults with and without depressive symptoms, considering gender and educational level. PeerJ. 2019 Apr 19;7:e6595. doi: 10.7717/peerj.6595. PMID: 31041148; PMCID: PMC6476293.

[36] Cabello R, Navarro Bravo B, Latorre JM, Fernández-Berrocal P. Ability of university-level education to prevent age-related decline in emotional intelligence. Front Aging Neurosci. 2014 Mar 11;6:37. doi: 10.3389/fnagi.2014.00037. PMID: 24653697; PMCID: PMC3949193.

[37] Brackett MA, Salovey P. Measuring emotional intelligence with the Mayer-Salovery-Caruso Emotional Intelligence Test (MSCEIT). Psicothema. 2006;18 Suppl:34-41. PMID: 17295955.

[38] Lim K, Lee SA, Pinkham AE, Lam M, Lee J. Evaluation of social cognitive measures in an Asian schizophrenia sample. Schizophr Res Cogn. 2019 Dec 10;20:100169. doi: 10.1016/j.scog.2019.100169. PMID: 32154121; PMCID: PMC7056931.

[39] Zhou Y. *Functional Neuroimaging with Multiple Modalities: Principle, Device and Applications*. Nova Science Publishers. 2016.

[40] Zhou Y. *Imaging and Multiomic Biomarker Applications: Advances in Early Alzheimer's Disease*. Nova Science Publishers. 2020.

[41] Zhou Y. J*oint Imaging Applications in General Neurodegenerative Disease: Parkinson's, Frontotemporal, Vascular Dementia and Autism*. Nova Science Publishers. 2021.

[42] Zhou Y. *Typical Imaging in Atypical Parkinson's, Schizophrenia, Epilepsy and Asymptomatic Alzheimer's Disease*. Nova Science Publishers. 2021.

[43] Megías A, Gutiérrez-Cobo MJ, Gómez-Leal R, Cabello R, Fernández-Berrocal P. Performance on emotional tasks engaging cognitive

control depends on emotional intelligence abilities: an ERP study. Sci Rep. 2017 Nov 27;7(1):16446. doi: 10.1038/s41598-017-16657-y. PMID: 29180769; PMCID: PMC5703978.

[44] Orzechowski J, Śmieja M, Lewczuk K, Nęcka E. Working memory updating of emotional stimuli predicts emotional intelligence in females. Sci Rep. 2020 Nov 30;10(1):20875. doi: 10.1038/s41598-020-77944-9. PMID: 33257769; PMCID: PMC7705704.

[45] Smith R, Lane RD, Alkozei A, Bao J, Smith C, Sanova A, Nettles M, Killgore WDS. Maintaining the feelings of others in working memory is associated with activation of the left anterior insula and left frontal-parietal control network. Soc Cogn Affect Neurosci. 2017 May 1;12(5):848-860. doi: 10.1093/scan/nsx011. PMID: 28158779; PMCID: PMC5460045)

[46] Habas C. Functional Connectivity of the Cognitive Cerebellum. Front Syst Neurosci. 2021 Apr 8;15:642225. doi: 10.3389/fnsys.2021. 642225. PMID: 33897382; PMCID: PMC8060696.

[47] Gutiérrez-Cobo MJ, Cabello R, Fernández-Berrocal P. Performance-based ability emotional intelligence benefits working memory capacity during performance on hot tasks. Sci Rep. 2017 Sep 15;7(1):11700. doi: 10.1038/s41598-017-12000-7. PMID: 28916754; PMCID: PMC5600979

[48] Demarin V, Bedeković MR, Puretić MB, Pašić MB. Arts, Brain and Cognition. Psychiatr Danub. 2016 Dec;28(4):343-348. PMID: 27855424.

[49] Stocco A, Sibert C, Steine-Hanson Z, Koh N, Laird JE, Lebiere CJ, Rosenbloom P. Analysis of the human connectome data supports the notion of a "Common Model of Cognition" for human and human-like intelligence across domains. Neuroimage. 2021 Jul 15;235:118035. doi: 10.1016/j.neuroimage.2021.118035. Epub 2021 Apr 7. PMID: 33838264.

[50] Beaty RE, Kenett YN, Christensen AP, Rosenberg MD, Benedek M, Chen Q, Fink A, Qiu J, Kwapil TR, Kane MJ, Silvia PJ. Robust prediction of individual creative ability from brain functional connectivity. Proc Natl Acad Sci U S A. 2018 Jan 30;115(5):1087-1092. doi: 10.1073/pnas.1713532115. Epub 2018 Jan 16. PMID: 29339474; PMCID: PMC5798342.

[51] Khalil R, Godde B, Karim AA. The Link Between Creativity, Cognition, and Creative Drives and Underlying Neural Mechanisms.

Front Neural Circuits. 2019 Mar 22;13:18. doi: 10.3389/fncir.2019. 00018. PMID: 30967763; PMCID: PMC6440443.

[52] Beaty RE, Benedek M, Silvia PJ, Schacter DL. Creative Cognition and Brain Network Dynamics. Trends Cogn Sci. 2016 Feb;20(2):87-95. doi: 10.1016/j.tics.2015.10.004. Epub 2015 Nov 6. PMID: 26553223; PMCID: PMC4724474.

[53] Beaty RE, Benedek M, Wilkins RW, Jauk E, Fink A, Silvia PJ, Hodges DA, Koschutnig K, Neubauer AC. Creativity and the default network: A functional connectivity analysis of the creative brain at rest. Neuropsychologia. 2014 Nov;64:92-8. doi: 10.1016/j.neuro psychologia.2014.09.019. Epub 2014 Sep 20. PMID: 25245940; PMCID: PMC4410786.

[54] Chen Q, Beaty RE, Wei D, Yang J, Sun J, Liu W, Yang W, Zhang Q, Qiu J. Longitudinal Alterations of Frontoparietal and Frontotemporal Networks Predict Future Creative Cognitive Ability. Cereb Cortex. 2018 Jan 1;28(1):103-115. doi: 10.1093/cercor/bhw353. PMID: 29253252.

[55] Patil AU, Madathil D, Huang CM. Healthy Aging Alters the Functional Connectivity of Creative Cognition in the Default Mode Network and Cerebellar Network. Front Aging Neurosci. 2021 Feb 18;13:607988. doi: 10.3389/fnagi.2021.607988. PMID: 33679372; PMCID: PMC7929978.

Chapter 4
Brain Changes Associated with Movies and Pictures

Abstract

The purpose of this chapter was to investigate both longitudinal session and conditional effects of fMRI paradigm including movie and flankers stimulation on brain, as well as the associated phenotypical correlations. With ICA-DR algorithm, both session and conditional effects were observed. For instance, during movie-watching, session-differences were reflected in the regions of medial orbitofrontal cortex, medial and superior frontal cortex, middle temporal gyrus, inferior parietal lobe, angular gyrus, motor/premotor area and visual cortex including subregions V1-V5, precuneus, cuneus, lingual, intracalcarine and occipital pole. Conditional network-based connectivity alterations such as movie vs. resting and inscape vs. resting comparisons involved mostly precuneus and inferior parietal gyrus. These dynamic network-based correlational changes indicated significant and specific visuo-motion enhancement of emotion/creativity/social communications that were related to the movie contents and brain cognitive processing. Significant functional network topological property with increased local and global network efficiencies (absolute) at later compared to earlier sessions for all conditions including movie and resting state were identified.

Significantly higher global VMHC Z-value during inscape stimulation compared to rest (P=0.02) and movie conditions (P=0.01) were observed. Global functional activity/conductivity z-value variations of each condition and session were exhibited additionally, such as relatively higher movie/inscape fALFF neural activity compared to rest/flankers conditions. Phenotypic associations were also revealed with fMRI metrics, including positive correlation between fALFF during movie watching condition and internal-state of hunger score as well as negative correlation between fALFF/VMHC global z-values during inscape stimulus and internal hunger/full scores. With dFNC connectogram analysis, similar distribution of mean dwell time of all six states in several sessions were observed with significantly lower mean dwell time in later session compared to baseline. Consistent with previous findings, our quantitative and multiparametric imaging results remained relatively consistent for different types of visual stimulations and tasks, suggesting temporal or long-term neuroplasticity and brain connectogram improvement from artistic and training paradigm such as movie and flankers.

Keywords: neuroplasticity, movie, inscape, flankers, task fMRI, movie paradigm, between-session variability, between-condition differences, visual cortex, arts perception, aesthetic, internal state, training effects, dynamic functional network connectivity, temporal dynamics, connectogram, dwell time, frequency, occupancy, visual cortex, angular gyrus, precuneus, cuneus, lingual, intracalcarine, occipital pole, medial orbitofrontal cortex, medial prefrontal cortex, superior frontal gyrus, emotion, creativity, social communications, brain network topology, long-term neuroplasticity

1. Introduction

Watching movie paradigm with fMRI could be used to improve brain function and characterize individual variation due to different contents, culture, background and environment [1]. Several issues had been addressed regarding the specific length and focused smooth activation patterns of movie fMRI, for the applications in neuroscience and neuropsychiatry. As an example, for the four conditions including movie/inscape/flankers/resting scanned over 12 times, across-session functional connectivity variation based on intraclass correlation coefficient metric was found to be greater than between-condition differences [2]. In other words, condition reliability or repeatability was high in frontoparietal and default mode networks (FPN and DMN), and comparable but slightly lower for between-session repeatability. The consistencies of different movie-watching functional connectivity patterns were further validated and connectivity results were predicted to be generalizable [3]. Also neural activity measured directly from magnetoencephalography (MEG) and reflected from blood oxygen-level dependent (BOLD) fMRI responses during movie viewing were in agreement mostly for the occipital cortex that also had strongest stimulus-dependent associations for each modality separately, followed by temporal and frontal lobes [4]. As for brain activation during video clip with naturalistic viewings, brain regions in the superior frontal area (BA6), inferior/superior parietal lobe together with DMN and insular/rolandic operculum were co-activated [5]. And during smooth pursuit in free movie viewing compared to saccades, middle cingulate extending to precuneus and temporoparietal junction had higher neural activities; while the superior temporal sulcus, inferior precuneus and supplementary eye field responded more to the background motion. These visuospatial capabilities suggested detectable prominent eye movements such as smooth pursuit besides saccade that involved more visual subregion V2 in the complex dynamic picture/movie watching situation [6]. Neural correlates of movie-enhanced emotional states such as surprise were exhibited in the DMN as high-level error monitoring center including the medial prefrontal node, in addition to the hippocampus and ventral striatum [7]. Also the sensorimotor cortex dynamic signal was specific to the temporally varying sensory events in a fine-grained manner, even during passive observation of movie [8]. Moreover, engagement with video stimuli such as preference and recall indicated neural similarity at temporal lobe and cerebellum that might be related to sensory integration and emotional processing [9]. Finally, classification accuracy including input imaging features from large regions of interest corresponding to visual naturalistic movie stimuli was higher and could be used to assess natural cognitive processing effects during movie watching [10].

The condition-specific functional connectivity fluctuations in the occipital and temporal regions during movie-watching were revealed, and reorganized more to the frontal and less to the parietal lobes based on dynamic and principle component analyses [11]. Also using synchronous fluctuation quantification, high inter-subject similarity coincided with lower network modularity and higher inter-network connectivity that were possibly due to more network integration and less segregation [12]. Dynamic functional connectivity increased in both ventral and dorsal visual streams with high stability during naturalistic movie watching together with the DMN (not the sensory-motor network) at resting state, while primary visual cortex stability was decreased under movie condition [13]. Distinguishable brain regions were involved regarding to different contents of the movie; for instance, medial and lateral prefrontal regions, frontal pole and posterior-inferior temporal/parietal/cingulate gyri as well as conventional amygdala exhibited lower activity, while longer frontal pole activation pattern existed for processing humor and novelty of the comedic events [14].

Viewing comedy movies in schizophrenia patients presented lower synchronous activity in the temporal, supramarginal and inferior parietal regions compared to controls, and clinical symptom correlated with the lower frontoparietal activity for humor processing in brain [15]. Also increased insular and attentional effective connectivity between cortical regions involved in attention and interoception as well as possible state switching disruption in melancholia during emotional film viewing had been reported [16]. Furthermore, adolescents with greater depressive symptoms presented atypical fMRI response such as dissimilarity to the rest of the group during movie viewing but similar item-level depressive profile including comparable corresponding brain activation patterns, while these changes were not present in depressive children [17].

The purpose of this chapter was to investigate both longitudinal session and conditional effects of fMRI paradigm including movie and flankers stimulation on brain together with associated phenotypical correlations. Inter-session differences of functional connectivity of typical networks and quantitative VMHC/ReHo/fALFF/topological efficiencies for neural activity/network correlation/conductivity were further examined, especially during movie-watching condition and were linked to the internal state behavioral scores.

2. Methods

2.1. Participants and Imaging Data

Imaging and phenotypic data were downloaded after approval from the website managed at NITRC and healthy brain network serial scanning initiative (HBN SSI) (http://fcon_1000.projects.nitrc. org/indi/IndiPro. html). Further information and some other DTI related and full-movie data were also available from the Child Mind Institute Healthy Brain Network (CMI-HBN), which shared the open science large-scale multimodal connectomics-based imaging dataset focusing on child and adolescent mental health and learning disorders [18-21]. Imaging data of 13 healthy adults (age range: 21-42, mean of 30.3 years) were scanned at 3T MRI repeatedly for 12 sessions acquired over 2 month periods, and four conditions were applied for each session. These four conditions included 10 minutes each of resting state (RS), naturalistic viewing of Inscape that consisted of moving abstract shapes with varying field-of-views, naturalistic viewing of movie clips from "Raiders of the Lost Arc" (Movie) and finally Flanker task. The orders of four conditions during each session were randomized and counter-balanced across the 12 sessions. MR data acquired with different orders were sorted and analyzed separately for each condition at each session to compare the differences and also evaluate test-retest reliabilities of fMRI data [22, 23].

2.2. Imaging Parameters and Data Processing

Four MRI experiments were performed using the 1.5T MRI scanner with standardized imaging protocols. The 3D MPRAGE sequence was run with TR/TI/TE=2730/1000/1.64 ms, flip angle=9°, matrix size=256 x 256 x 176, resolution=1 x 1x 1 mm^3 for reference image used in RS-fMRI activity/connectivity/conductivity maps, as well as for structural morphological analysis. For the resting-state (RS)-fMRI data acquired, a standard gradient-echo EPI sequence (TR/TE=1450/40 msec, number of volumes=420, spatial resolution=2.5 x 2.5 x 2.5 mm^3) was utilized [2].

The MRI and fMRI images at baseline and four longitudinal sessions with equal intervals including session numbers of 2, 6 10 and 14 acquired over 2 month periods were re-ordered and post-processed with the in-house developed scripts to derive the VMHC, VBM, ICA-DR, ReHo map, graph theory based small-worldness systematic analysis and dFNC, using the similar methods described in previous chapters and our recent works [24]. Correlations between functional quantitative MRI metrics such as fALFF/VMHC/ReHo and phenotypic data such as internal state questionnaire of hungry, thirst and full scales before and after scan (ISQ and ISQ2 respectively) were also performed to examine the associations between imaging and behavior/neural cognitive metrics under four conditions including movie watching.

3. Results

Significant between-session differences (with total of four) in movie-related network connectivity were presented in Figure 1 A-C

(P<0.001), with relatively larger between-session differences compared to between-condition results. Regions in the medial orbitofrontal cortex, medial and superior frontal cortex, middle temporal gyrus, inferior parietal lobe, angular gyrus, motor/premotor area, primary visual cortex subregions V1-V5, lateral occipital clusters including precuneus, cuneus, lingual, intracalcarine and occipital pole showed significant and specific longitudinal visuo-motion enhancement and emotion/creativity/ social interaction network connections during movie watching. Figure 1D showed differences between conditions such as movie vs. resting and inscape vs. resting comparisons, with mostly precuneus and inferior parietal gyrus involved. Figure 2 presented functional network topological property changes during movie watching with increased local and global network efficiencies (absolute) at later compared to earlier sessions. Similar functional network topological property changes during resting condition were observed including higher local and global network efficiencies (absolute) at later sessions as shown in Figure 3. Network sparsity level increased compared movie to resting conditions, possibly due to slightly higher local efficiency with movie watching stimulation (Figure 3). In contrast to the between-session differences, functional network topological properties under four conditions were almost identical for all sessions, and representative early session 2 (SSV2) was illustrated in Figure 4. Also Figure 5 illustrated close functional network topological properties under four conditions at end session 14 (SSV14).

Evaluations of global quantitative fALFF Z-values and sub-bands S4/S5 changes during four different conditions (Rest, Inscape, Movie and Flankers in Figure 6A) at different sessions (SSV2-SSV14 in Figure 6B) were performed. Variations of each condition and session could be observed, such as relatively higher movie/inscape fALFF neural activity compared to rest/flankers conditions and relatively higher activity at sessions SSV6 and SSV10. There were no significant statistical differences between sessions and conditions for all global fALFF comparisons. Figure 7 showed comparison of VMHC global Z-values during four types of conditions (Rest, Inscape, Movie and Flankers) at different sessions (SSV2-SSV14) as well. Significantly higher VMHC Z-value during inscape stimulation compared to both rest (P=0.02) and movie (P=0.01) were discovered for the between-condition difference comparisons. Larger VMHC values at later sessions were also observed compared to early ones, including both inscape stimulation (SSV14 vs. SSV10, P=0.01) and movie condition (P=0.01 comparing session SSV6 to SSV2; P=0.002 comparing SSV14 to SSV2 and P=0.04 comparing SSV14 to SSV10). No other significant voxel-wise VMHC or fALFF or ReHo differences between-condition or between session were found with P>0.05.

Significant correlations ($|r|>0.62$, P<0.05) between fMRI fALFF/VMHC global Z-values and phenotypic score of ISQ measuring full, hunger and thirst states were displayed in Figure 8. Strong associations between global Z-value of fALFF (full band and lower band S5) during movie watching condition and ISQ/ISQ2 hunger score were observed. On the other hand, only negative associations between fALFF/VMHC global z-values during inscape and ISQ/ISQ2 hunger or full scores existed as well. Quantitative results between two metrics are listed as:

1). Movie fALFF S4 and ISQ2 Hunger, r=-0.7205, P=0.0285;
2). Inscape fALFF S4 and ISQ2 Full, r=-0.6925, P=0.0264;
3). Inscape fALFF S4 and ISQ Hunger, r=-0.6382, P=0.0471;
4). Movie fALFF S5 and ISQ Hunger, r=0.6865, P=0.0411;
5). Inscape fALFF S5 and ISQ Full, r=-0.7260, P=0.0414;
6). Movie fALFF S5 and ISQ2 Full, r=-0.6322, P=0.0499;
7). Movie fALFF and ISQ Hunger, r=0.7973, P=0.0178;
8). Movie fALFF and ISQ2 Hunger, r=0.7185, P=0.0446;

9). Inscape VMHC and ISQ2 Hunger, r=-0.6216, P=0.041.

Figure 9 demonstrated the distribution of dynamic dwell time in each of the six states for four longitudinal sessions based on the dFNC analysis, with evenly distribution of number of occurrences at each state in session SSV10 and slightly less dynamics at end session. Bar plots of mean dwell time and fractional occupancy of six states in different sessions showed significantly lower mean dwell time in session SSV10 compared to baseline SSV1 with P=0.037 (Figure 10). Similar distributions of dwell time of all six states in three sessions of SSV1, SSV2 and SSV6 were indicated in Figure 11. The distribution pattern of mean dwell time in SSV14 was different than all the previous sessions with bi-modal peaks compared to the single peak distribution of all earlier four sessions including baseline (Figure 12).

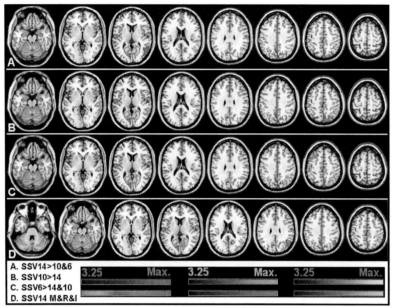

Figure 1. *Significant session (A-C) and stimulus effects in movie-related intra- and inter-network connectivity (P<0.001) including the DMN, frontal CEN, MN, VN and FPN. Regions in the medial orbitofrontal cortex, medial and superior frontal cortex, middle temporal gyrus, inferior parietal lobe, angular gyrus, motor/premotor area, visual cortex subregions V1-V5, occipital lobe including precuneus, cuneus, lingual, intracalcarine and occipital pole showed significant and specific visuo-motion enhancement and emotion/creativity/social interaction network connections during movie watching at latter sessions. Panel D showed differences between conditions such as movie vs. resting and inscape vs. resting, with mostly precuneus and inferior parietal gyrus involved.*

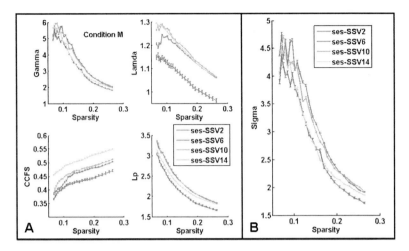

Figure 2. *Functional network topological property changes during movie watching: increased local and global network efficiencies (absolute) at later sessions compared to earlier ones.*

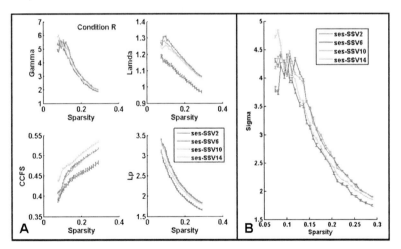

Figure 3. *Similar functional network topological property changes during resting condition (condition R): increased local and global network efficiencies (absolute) at later sessions. Compared movie to resting conditions, network sparsity level increased, possibly due to slightly higher local efficiency during movie watching stimulation.*

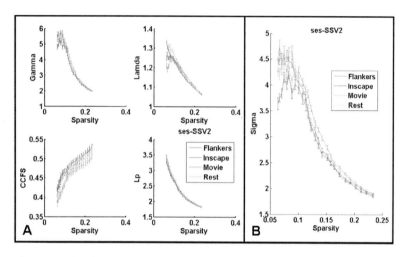

Figure 4. *Close functional network topological properties under four conditions at initial session SSV2.*

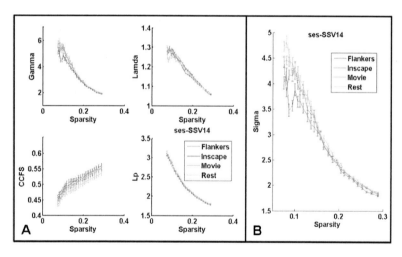

Figure 5. *Close functional network topological properties under four conditions at end session SSV14.*

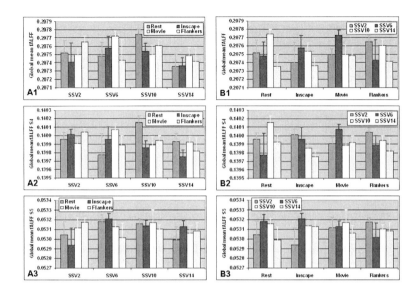

Figure 6. *Evaluation of fALFF and sub-bands S4/S5 changes (panel 1-3 respectively) during four different conditions (Rest, Inscape, Movie and Flankers in A) at different sessions (SSV2-SSV14 in B). Variations of each condition and session could be observed, such as relatively higher movie/inscape fALFF neural activity compared to rest/flankers conditions and relatively higher activity at session SSV6 and SSV10. There were no significant statistical differences between sessions and conditions for all six subplot comparisons.*

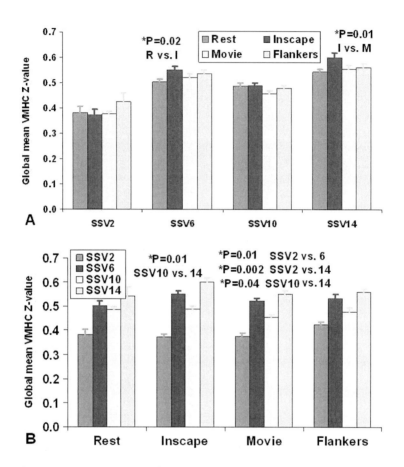

Figure 7. A: *Comparison of VMHC global Z-values during four different conditions (Rest, Inscape, Movie and Flankers) at different sessions (SSV2-SSV14). Significantly higher between-condition VMHC Z-value during inscape stimulation compared to rest (P=0.02) and higher VMHC compared inscape to movie conditions as well (P=0.01) were observed. B: Significantly higher between-session VMHC at later sessions compared to early ones during inscape (SSV10 vs. SSV14, P=0.01) and movie condition (P=0.01 comparing SSV6 to SSV2; P=0.002 comparing SSV14 to SSV2 and P=0.04 comparing SSV14 to SSV10).*

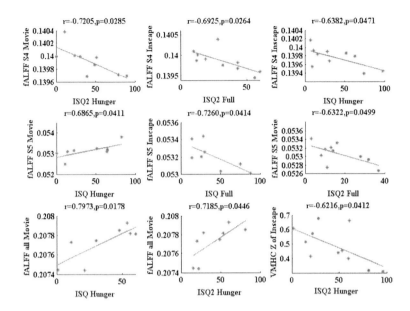

Figure 8. *Significant correlations ($|r|>0.62$, $P<0.05$) between fMRI fALFF/VMHC global Z-values and phenotypic score of internal state questionnaire ISQ & ISQ2 measuring full, hunger and thirst. Strong positive associations between fALFF (full band and lower band S5) global Z-value of movie watching condition and ISQ hunger score were observed. On the other hand, negative associations between fALFF and VMHC global z-values during inscape and ISQ hunger or full scores existed as well.*

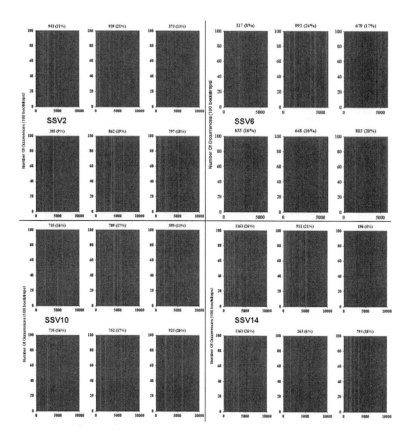

Figure 9. *Distribution of dynamic dwell time in each of the six states for four longitudinal sessions based on the dFNC analysis. Evenly distributions for number of occurrences at each state (in the range of 13%-20%) in session SSV10 were observed, with slightly less dynamics at end session.*

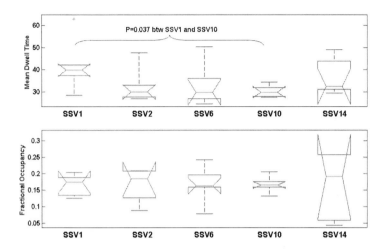

Figure 10. *Barplots of mean dwell time and fractional occupancy of six states in different sessions. Significantly lower mean dwell time in session SSV10 compared to baseline SSV1 with P=0.037. No other between-session differences of mean dwell time or frequency existed with P>0.05.*

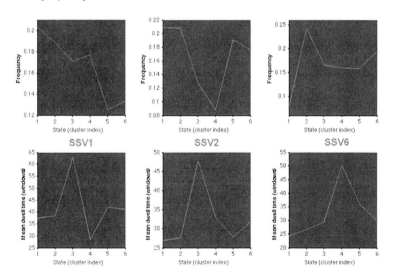

Figure 11. *Similar distribution of mean dwell time of all six states in three sessions SSV1, SSV2 and SSV6.*

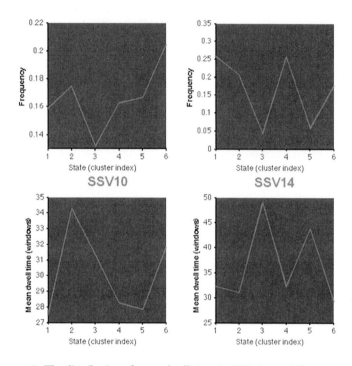

Figure 12. *The distribution of mean dwell time in SSV14 was different than all the previous sessions with bi-modal peaks compared to the single peak distribution of all earlier four sampled sessions. Pattern of dwell time in SSV10 was similar to previous SSV1-SSV6 patterns in Figure 11.*

4. Discussion

4.1. Summary of Results

With ICA-DR algorithm, both session and conditional effects were observed for multiple intra- and inter- network connectivities and relatively larger between-session difference compared to between-condition variation were revealed. For instance, session-differences during movie-watching were reflected in the regions of medial orbitofrontal cortex, medial and superior frontal cortex, middle temporal gyrus, inferior parietal lobe, angular gyrus, motor/

premotor area, visual cortex including V1-V5, occipital clusters including precuneus, cuneus, lingual, intracalcarine and occipital pole. Conditional network-based connectivity alterations such as movie vs. resting and inscape vs. resting comparisons involved mostly precuneus and inferior parietal gyrus. These dynamic network-based correlational changes indicated significant and specific visuo-motion enhancement and emotion/creativity/ social interactions that were possibly related to the movie contents and brain cognitive processing. Based on graph theory implemented to the functional connectivity data, detectable between-session differences could also be observed but with quite close between-condition parameters. Furthermore, significant functional network topological property with increased local and global network efficiencies (absolute) at later sessions compared to earlier sessions in all four conditions including movie and resting state were identified.

For global functional quantification, significantly higher VMHC Z-value during inscape stimulation compared to rest (P=0.02) and movie conditions (P=0.01) were observed. No other significant between-condition or between-session differences of VMHC were found with P>0.05. For ReHo and fALFF, there were no significant statistical differences between sessions and conditions. Slight variations of fALFF/ReHo metrics among different condition and session could be observed, such as relatively higher movie/inscape fALFF neural activity compared to rest/flankers conditions and relatively higher activity at middle sessions of SSV6 and SSV10. Phenotypic associations were observed between fMRI metrics, including positive correlation between fALFF during movie watching condition and ISQ hunger score before and after scans as well as negative correlation between fALFF/VMHC global z-values during inscape stimulus and ISQ hunger/full scores.

With dFNC connectogram analysis, similar distribution of mean dwell time of all six states in three sessions of SSV1, SSV2 and SSV6 were observed. Significantly lower mean dwell time in session SSV10 compared to baseline SSV1 existed, and the distribution of dwell time in SSV14 was different than all the previous sessions with bi-modal peaks compared to the single peak distribution of all earlier four sessions.

4.2. Summary of Related Imaging Findings

4.2.1 Visual Perception and Pathway in Brain

The inferior parietal sulcus (IPS) activation for object-motion isolation and perceptual integration processing were found to modulate the early visual area responses by fast global template extraction and efficient visual inputs direction for the first impression such as within the early 100 ms [25, 26]. As expected, the visual attention areas in response to the natural scene viewing (such as painting or passively watching movie) for object localization were enhanced along the visuospatial attention-salient elements pathway for projection and information allocation [27]. And the primary visual cortex V1 and V2 areas played important roles in both elementary visual features and fine representations of natural scene that were joined and represented further in the higher-level visual processing including V4 for color mapping and V3/V5 for global motion detection and pattern integration [28, 29]. The low and mid-level or intermediate stages corresponding to visual scene perception, pattern information and initial semantic processing utilized multimodal analysis such as both visual and auditory contribution that occurred more in the posterior ventral temporal cortex in addition to the early visual areas and multi-layer visual regions as well as occipitotemporal junction [30]. Moreover, the neural activity pattern in the hippocampus differentiated between episodic elements including people, locations and narrative contents such as stories, forming the spatial map encoding for short-term narrative-context representation and memory consolidation [31]. And the dorsomedial prefrontal cortex (DMPFC) was found to be involved in social interactions between playing characters, while the co-varied regions including inferior parietal and temporal areas were specifically tuned to faces and actions [32]. The brain basis for these complex social communications shared similar consciousness state and inter-subject neural synchronization [33].

4.2.2 Visual Arts including Writing/Calligraphy/Painting Related Neuroimaging Findings

Writing-specific regions including superior/middle frontal gyri, intra-parietal sulcus/superior parietal area and cerebellum in addition to the general motor functional areas such as sensorimotor/supplementary motor/motor and subcortical striatum were discovered during handwriting experiment with neuroimaging techniques [34]. Also visual perception of complexity for artistic images and mathematical fractals centered more within the relatively high alpha and beta bands in the occipitoparietal regions, and the parietal alpha power reflected neural substrates for complex stimuli [35]. Gray matter volume in the right precuneus and posterior cingulate cortex for long-term Chinese calligraphic handwriting (CCH) was reduced, and was associated with attention and meditation [36]. Moreover, the executive control network from resting-state functional connectivity and corresponding cognitive function of inhibition and updating were improved with long-term CCH [37]. The global and local efficiencies of brain network topological configuration in the frontoparietal network, basal ganglia, subcortical thalamus and limbic system were increased in the CCH group compared to controls [38]. Further, enhanced activations for possible aesthetic experience in the superior parietal lobe, anterior cingulate and insula were identified comparing conditions of watching the creation of calligraphy image to no observation [39]. Also increased activations of premotor/motor areas as well as orbitofrontal and prefrontal areas were reported during observation of abstract paintings, possibly for detailed cortical appreciation of static meaningless art and reward perception [40]. Using effective connectivity analysis, the ventral striatum was driven by the visual signal when viewing art but not by non-art images, regardless of individual esthetic preferences [41]. Increased connectivity between visual cortex sub-region V4 and ventro-lateral prefrontal cortex during color naming as well as higher gray matter activation were discovered in painting-major individuals compared to non-majors [42]. In addition, narrative comprehension linked brain networks such as DMN for simulating features and behavior dynamically, as well as the somatomotor, visual and ventral attention functional connectivity systems that were sensitive to movie and intermediate low-demand pattern video such as inscape conditions compared to resting state [43, 44]. Taken together, viewing painting arts engaged several systems such as occipital and temporal lobes for visual representation and object/scene recognition, ventral striatum and orbitofrontal cortex/hypothalamus for reward perception as well as posterior cingulate cortex in the DMN and insular structure for emotional experience and internalized cognitions [45].

4.2.3 Aesthetic Perception Related Findings

Several brain regions and systems were related to the aesthetic perception or artistic work assessments, including the dorsolateral prefrontal cortex (DLPFC), medial orbitofrontal cortex (mOFC) and insula. For instance, anterior insula was reported to be activated for aesthetic appraisal of artworks for the social needs and psychological satisfaction, and the prefrontal white matter neuroplasticity change reflected creativity gain in the art students compared to non-art controls [46, 47]. Also the mOFC activity was enhanced during the experience of musical and visual beauty, while the DLPFC played critical role for aesthetic appreciation of paintings and photographs [48, 49]. In addition to the valuation modulation of ventromedial prefrontal cortex (vmPFC), DLPFC had also been revealed to control cognitive and emotion responses by removing the monetary favors (executive function and appreciation role against other judgment bias) in response to the art-viewing task with reward incentive paradigm [50]. Greater functional integration of the DMN as well as environmentally driven attention control of the salience and attentional neural networks (SN) during movie watching in adulthood predicted the fluid intelligence in the way that stronger expression of communication profile with essential element variability and information related to higher intelligence [51].

4.2.4 Movie and Arts Therapy

In children with autism compared to typically developed children, less synchrony in the social cognition regions (related to theory of mind) such as mOFC, temporoparietal junction and lateral prefrontal cortex were reported, together with the abnormal functional integration and segregation during movie-watching [52, 53]. Applications of fMRI in several major psychiatric disorders had achieved great success and involved several advanced topics such as fine experiment paradigm and improved disease classifications together with integrative protocol of genetic, phenotypic and multiomic data for better pathophysiological interpretation [54]. Specifically, functional connectome for intra- and inter- network correlational quantification identified hyper-connectivity between DMN, salience and attentional networks (SN) in youth with attention-deficit and hyperactivity disorder (ADHD) [55]. In schizophrenia, distributed network alterations with functionally disconnected star nodes in brain were in agreement with the psychosis hypothesis based on computational connectomics [56]. And in first-episode psychosis patients, less correlation between precuneal function and movie fantasy contents was found compared to controls with ~80% disease classification accuracy including positive symptom score [57]. Moreover, several studies had also investigated the contribution from movie paradigm of social cognition for better understanding of neural mechanisms in anxiety and autism disorders, as well as applying advanced connectome-based models to predict participant's phenotypic assessments such as processing speed, memory and attention in aging [58]. The fMRI inter-subject correlations (ISC) were higher in the DMN for ADHD but weaker in attentional network compared to controls, during the post-scan recall of a multi-talker film with auditory background distraction [59]. Aside from ISC, revealing network interactions during complex naturalistic conditions and dynamic longitudinal connectome alteration to quantify movie-watching connectivity changes relative to resting state and conventional tasks hold certain potentials in pediatric and neurodevelopmental disorder applications [60].

4.3. Conclusion

In conclusion, both session and condition effects were observed such as watching inscape and movie; including relatively larger between-session differences in distinct visual areas such as V1-V5 as well as lingual and precuneus for significant and specific longitudinal visuo-motion enhancement of emotion/creativity/ social communication that were in response to the movie contents, visual perception and cognitive processing. Functional global quantification of neural activity and interhemispheric correlation values were associated with internal state scores of hungry and full scale before and after scans. Increased local and global efficiencies of later session compared to earlier ones for all four conditions indicated improvement of neural resource utilization after training and knowledge buildup. Our multiparametric imaging quantification results were consistent with previously reported findings, and emphasized the fine detailed and specific brain regional activations in visual arts and aesthetic evaluation as well as visual insight profits during movie/picture viewing. And these results remained relatively consistent for different types of visual stimulations and tasks, suggesting temporal or long-term neuroplasticity and brain connectogram improvement from artistic and training fMRI paradigms.

References

[1] Eickhoff SB, Milham M, Vanderwal T. Towards clinical applications of movie fMRI. Neuroimage. 2020 Aug 15;217:116860. doi: 10.1016/j.neuroimage.2020.116860. Epub 2020 May 4. PMID: 32376301.

[2] O'Connor D, Potler NV, Kovacs M, Xu T, Ai L, Pellman J, Vanderwal T, Parra LC, Cohen S, Ghosh S, Escalera J, Grant-Villegas N, Osman Y, Bui A, Craddock RC, Milham MP. The Healthy Brain Network Serial Scanning Initiative: a resource for evaluating inter-individual differences and their reliabilities across scan conditions and sessions. Gigascience. 2017 Feb 1;6(2):1-14. doi: 10.1093/gigascience/giw011. PMID: 28369458; PMCID: PMC5466711.

[3] Tian L, Ye M, Chen C, Cao X, Shen T. Consistency of functional connectivity across different movies. Neuroimage. 2021 Jun;233:117926. doi: 10.1016/j.neuroimage.2021.117926. Epub 2021 Mar 3. PMID: 33675997.

[4] Lankinen K, Saari J, Hlushchuk Y, Tikka P, Parkkonen L, Hari R, Koskinen M. Consistency and similarity of MEG- and fMRI-signal time courses during movie viewing. Neuroimage. 2018 Jun;173:361-369. doi: 10.1016/j.neuroimage.2018.02.045. Epub 2018 Feb 24. PMID: 29486325.

[5] Kim HC, Jin S, Jo S, Lee JH. A naturalistic viewing paradigm using 360° panoramic video clips and real-time field-of-view changes with eye-gaze tracking. Neuroimage. 2020 Aug 1;216:116617. doi: 10.1016/j.neuroimage.2020.116617. Epub 2020 Feb 10. PMID: 32057996.

[6] Agtzidis I, Meyhöfer I, Dorr M, Lencer R. Following Forrest Gump: Smooth pursuit related brain activation during free movie viewing. Neuroimage. 2020 Aug 1;216:116491. doi: 10.1016/j.neuroimage.2019.116491. Epub 2020 Jan 7. PMID: 31923604.

[7] Brandman T, Malach R, Simony E. The surprising role of the default mode network in naturalistic perception. Commun Biol. 2021 Jan 19;4(1):79. doi: 10.1038/s42003-020-01602-z. PMID: 33469113; PMCID: PMC7815915.

[8] Lankinen K, Smeds E, Tikka P, Pihko E, Hari R, Koskinen M. Haptic contents of a movie dynamically engage the spectator's sensorimotor cortex. Hum Brain Mapp. 2016 Nov;37(11):4061-4068. doi: 10.1002/hbm.23295. PMID: 27364184; PMCID: PMC5108418.

[9] Chan HY, Smidts A, Schoots VC, Dietvorst RC, Boksem MAS. Neural similarity at temporal lobe and cerebellum predicts out-of-sample preference and recall for video stimuli. Neuroimage. 2019 Aug 15;197:391-401. doi: 10.1016/j.neuroimage.2019.04.076. Epub 2019 May 1. PMID: 31051296.

[10] Mandelkow H, de Zwart JA, Duyn JH. Linear Discriminant Analysis Achieves High Classification Accuracy for the BOLD fMRI Response to Naturalistic Movie Stimuli. Front Hum Neurosci. 2016 Mar 31;10:128. doi: 10.3389/fnhum.2016.00128. PMID: 27065832; PMCID: PMC4815557.

[11] Demirtaş M, Ponce-Alvarez A, Gilson M, Hagmann P, Mantini D, Betti V, Romani GL, Friston K, Corbetta M, Deco G. Distinct modes of functional connectivity induced by movie-watching. Neuroimage. 2019 Jan 1;184:335-348. doi: 10.1016/j.neuroimage.2018.09.042. Epub 2018 Sep 17. PMID: 30237036; PMCID: PMC6248881.

[12] Betzel RF, Byrge L, Esfahlani FZ, Kennedy DP. Temporal fluctuations in the brain's modular architecture during movie-watching. Neuroimage. 2020 Jun;213:116687. doi: 10.1016/j.neuroimage. 2020.116687. Epub 2020 Feb 29. PMID: 32126299; PMCID: PMC7165071.

[13] Li L, Lu B, Yan CG. Stability of dynamic functional architecture differs between brain networks and states. Neuroimage. 2020 Aug 1;216:116230. doi: 10.1016/j.neuroimage.2019.116230. Epub 2019 Sep 29. PMID: 31577959.

[14] Jääskeläinen IP, Pajula J, Tohka J, Lee HJ, Kuo WJ, Lin FH. Brain hemodynamic activity during viewing and re-viewing of comedy movies explained by experienced humor. Sci Rep. 2016 Jun 21;6:27741. doi: 10.1038/srep27741. PMID: 27323928; PMCID: PMC4914983.

[15] Tu PC, Su TP, Lin WC, Chang WC, Bai YM, Li CT, Lin FH. Reduced synchronized brain activity in schizophrenia during viewing of comedy movies. Sci Rep. 2019 Sep 4;9(1):12738. doi: 10.1038/s41598-019-48957-w. PMID: 31484998; PMCID: PMC6726596.

[16] Hyett MP, Parker GB, Guo CC, Zalesky A, Nguyen VT, Yuen T, Breakspear M. Scene unseen: Disrupted neuronal adaptation in melancholia during emotional film viewing. Neuroimage Clin. 2015 Oct 24;9:660-7. doi: 10.1016/j.nicl.2015.10.011. PMID: 26740919; PMCID: PMC4660155.

[17] Gruskin DC, Rosenberg MD, Holmes AJ. Relationships between depressive symptoms and brain responses during emotional movie viewing emerge in adolescence. Neuroimage. 2020 Aug 1;216:116217. doi: 10.1016/j.neuroimage.2019.116217. Epub 2019 Oct 16. PMID: 31628982; PMCID: PMC7958984.

[18] Vanderwal T, Kelly C, Eilbott J, Mayes LC, Castellanos FX. Inscapes: A movie paradigm to improve compliance in functional magnetic resonance imaging. Neuroimage. 2015 Nov 15;122:222-32. doi: 10.1016/j.neuroimage.2015.07.069. Epub 2015 Aug 1. PMID: 26241683; PMCID: PMC4618190.

[19] Betti V, Della Penna S, de Pasquale F, Mantini D, Marzetti L, Romani GL, Corbetta M. Natural scenes viewing alters the dynamics of functional connectivity in the human brain. Neuron. 2013 Aug 21;79(4):782-97. doi: 10.1016/j.neuron.2013.06.022. Epub 2013 Jul 25. PMID: 23891400; PMCID: PMC3893318.

[20] Ulrich R, Prislan L, Miller J. A bimodal extension of the Eriksen flanker task. Atten Percept Psychophys. 2021 Feb;83(2):790-799. doi: 10.3758/s13414-020-02150-8. Epub 2020 Nov 11. PMID: 33179215; PMCID: PMC7884581.

[21] Di X, Biswal BB. Intersubject consistent dynamic connectivity during natural vision revealed by functional MRI. Neuroimage. 2020 Aug 1;216:116698. doi: 10.1016/j.neuroimage.2020.116698. Epub 2020 Mar 1. PMID: 32130972.

[22] Alexander LM, Escalera J, Ai L, Andreotti C, Febre K, Mangone A, Vega-Potler N, Langer N, Alexander A, Kovacs M, Litke S, O'Hagan B, Andersen J, Bronstein B, Bui A, Bushey M, Butler H, Castagna V, Camacho N, Chan E, Citera D, Clucas J, Cohen S, Dufek S, Eaves M, Fradera B, Gardner J, Grant-Villegas N, Green G, Gregory C, Hart E, Harris S, Horton M, Kahn D, Kabotyanski K, Karmel B, Kelly SP, Kleinman K, Koo B, Kramer E, Lennon E, Lord C, Mantello G, Margolis A, Merikangas KR, Milham J, Minniti G, Neuhaus R, Levine A, Osman Y, Parra LC, Pugh KR, Racanello A, Restrepo A, Saltzman T, Septimus B, Tobe R, Waltz R, Williams A, Yeo A, Castellanos FX, Klein A, Paus T, Leventhal BL, Craddock RC, Koplewicz HS, Milham MP. An open resource for transdiagnostic research in pediatric mental health and learning disorders. Sci Data. 2017 Dec 19;4:170181. doi: 10.1038/sdata.2017.181. PMID: 29257126; PMCID: PMC5735921.

[23] Zuo XN, Xu T, Milham MP. Harnessing reliability for neuroscience research. Nat Hum Behav. 2019 Aug;3(8):768-771. doi: 10.1038/s41562-019-0655-x. PMID: 31253883.

[24] Zhou Y. *Typical Imaging in Atypical Parkinson's, Schizophrenia, Epilepsy and Asymptomatic Alzheimer's Disease.* Nova Science Publishers. 2021.

[25] Liu L, Wang F, Zhou K, Ding N, Luo H. Perceptual integration rapidly activates dorsal visual pathway to guide local processing in early visual areas. PLoS Biol. 2017 Nov 30;15(11):e2003646. doi: 10.1371/journal.pbio.2003646. PMID: 29190640; PMCID: PMC5726727;

[26] Field DT, Biagi N, Inman LA. The role of the ventral intraparietal area (VIP/pVIP) in the perception of object-motion and self-motion. Neuroimage. 2020 Jun;213:116679. doi: 10.1016/j.neuroimage.2020.116679. Epub 2020 Feb 26. PMID: 32112961.

[27] Zipser K. Visualizing fMRI BOLD responses to diverse naturalistic scenes using retinotopic projection. J Vis. 2017 Jun 1;17(6):18. doi: 10.1167/17.6.18. PMID: 28654963.

[28] Farivar R, Clavagnier S, Hansen BC, Thompson B, Hess RF. Non-uniform phase sensitivity in spatial frequency maps of the human visual cortex. J Physiol. 2017 Feb 15;595(4):1351-1363. doi: 10.1113/JP273206. Epub 2017 Feb 2. PMID: 27748961; PMCID: PMC5309370.;

[29] Movshon JA, Simoncelli EP. Representation of Naturalistic Image Structure in the Primate Visual Cortex. Cold Spring Harb Symp Quant Biol. 2014;79:115-22. doi: 10.1101/sqb.2014.79.024844. Epub 2015 May 5. PMID: 25943766; PMCID: PMC4800008.

[30] Groen II, Silson EH, Baker CI. Integrated deep visual and semantic attractor neural networks predict fMRI pattern-information along the ventral object processing pathway; Contributions of low- and high-level properties to neural processing of visual scenes in the human brain. Philos Trans R Soc Lond B Biol Sci. 2017 Feb 19;372(1714):20160102. doi: 10.1098/rstb.2016.0102. Epub 2017 Jan 2. PMID: 28044013; PMCID: PMC5206270.

[31] Milivojevic B, Varadinov M, Vicente Grabovetsky A, Collin SH, Doeller CF. Coding of Event Nodes and Narrative Context in the Hippocampus. J Neurosci. 2016 Dec 7;36(49):12412-12424. doi: 10.1523/JNEUROSCI.2889-15.2016. Erratum in: J Neurosci. 2017 May 31;37(22):5588. PMID: 27927958; PMCID: PMC6601969.

[32] Wagner DD, Kelley WM, Haxby JV, Heatherton TF. The Dorsal Medial Prefrontal Cortex Responds Preferentially to Social Interactions during Natural Viewing. J Neurosci. 2016 Jun 29;36(26):6917-25. doi: 10.1523/JNEUROSCI.4220-15.2016. PMID: 27358450; PMCID: PMC4926239.

[33] Nummenmaa L, Lahnakoski JM, Glerean E. Sharing the social world via intersubject neural synchronisation. Curr Opin Psychol. 2018 Dec;24:7-14. doi: 10.1016/j.copsyc.2018.02.021. Epub 2018 Mar 8. PMID: 29550395.

[34] Planton S, Jucla M, Roux FE, Démonet JF. The "handwriting brain": a meta-analysis of neuroimaging studies of motor versus orthographic processes. Cortex. 2013 Nov-Dec;49(10):2772-87. doi: 10.1016/j.cortex. 2013.05.011. Epub 2013 Jun 12. PMID: 23831432.

[35] Rawls E, White R, Kane S, Stevens CE Jr, Zabelina DL. Parametric Cortical Representations of Complexity and Preference for Artistic and Computer-Generated Fractal Patterns Revealed by Single-Trial EEG Power Spectral Analysis. Neuroimage. 2021 Aug 1;236:118092. doi: 10.1016/j.neuroimage.2021.118092. Epub 2021 Apr 23. PMID: 33895307; PMCID: PMC8287964.

[36] Chen W, Chen C, Yang P, Bi S, Liu J, Xia M, Lin Q, Ma N, Li N, He Y, Zhang J, Wang Y, Wang W. Long-term Chinese calligraphic handwriting reshapes the posterior cingulate cortex: A VBM study. PLoS One. 2019 Apr 4;14(4):e0214917. doi: 10.1371/journal.pone. 0214917. PMID: 30947247; PMCID: PMC6448813.

[37] Chen W, He Y, Gao Y, Zhang C, Chen C, Bi S, Yang P, Wang Y, Wang W. Long-Term Experience of Chinese Calligraphic Handwriting Is Associated with Better Executive Functions and Stronger Resting-State Functional Connectivity in Related Brain Regions. PLoS One. 2017 Jan 27;12(1):e0170660. doi: 10.1371/journal.pone.0170660. PMID: 28129407; PMCID: PMC5271317.

[38] Chen W, He Y, Chen C, Zhu M, Bi S, Liu J, Xia M, Lin Q, Wang Y, Wang W. Long-term Chinese calligraphic handwriting training has a positive effect on brain network efficiency. PLoS One. 2019 Jan 25;14(1):e0210962. doi: 10.1371/journal.pone.0210962. PMID: 30682084; PMCID: PMC6347361.

[39] He M, Zhang W, Deng J, He X. The effect of action observation on aesthetic preference of Chinese calligraphy: An fMRI study. Brain

Behav. 2021 Aug;11(8):e2265. doi: 10.1002/brb3.2265. Epub 2021 Jun 21. PMID: 34152097; PMCID: PMC8413759.

[40] Sbriscia-Fioretti B, Berchio C, Freedberg D, Gallese V, Umiltà MA. ERP modulation during observation of abstract paintings by Franz Kline. PLoS One. 2013 Oct 9;8(10):e75241. doi: 10.1371/journal.pone. 0075241. PMID: 24130693; PMCID: PMC3793982.

[41] Lacey S, Hagtvedt H, Patrick VM, Anderson A, Stilla R, Deshpande G, Hu X, Sato JR, Reddy S, Sathian K. Art for reward's sake: visual art recruits the ventral striatum. Neuroimage. 2011 Mar 1;55(1):420-33. doi: 10.1016/j.neuroimage. 2010.11.027. Epub 2010 Nov 25. PMID: 21111833; PMCID: PMC3031763.

[42] Long Z, Peng D, Chen K, Jin Z, Yao L. Neural substrates in color processing: a comparison between painting majors and non-majors. Neurosci Lett. 2011 Jan 7;487(2):191-5. doi: 10.1016/j.neulet. 2010.10.020. Epub 2010 Oct 15. PMID: 20951765.

[43] Simony E, Honey CJ, Chen J, Lositsky O, Yeshurun Y, Wiesel A, Hasson U. Dynamic reconfiguration of the default mode network during narrative comprehension. Nat Commun. 2016 Jul 18;7:12141. doi: 10.1038/ncomms12141. PMID: 27424918; PMCID: PMC4960303.

[44] Vanderwal T, Kelly C, Eilbott J, Mayes LC, Castellanos FX. Inscapes: A movie paradigm to improve compliance in functional magnetic resonance imaging. Neuroimage. 2015 Nov 15;122:222-32. doi: 10.1016/j.neuroimage.2015.07.069. Epub 2015 Aug 1. PMID: 26241683; PMCID: PMC4618190.

[45] Vartanian O, Skov M. Neural correlates of viewing paintings: evidence from a quantitative meta-analysis of functional magnetic resonance imaging data. Brain Cogn. 2014 Jun;87:52-6. doi: 10.1016/j.bandc. 2014.03.004. Epub 2014 Apr 4. PMID: 24704947.

[46] Brown S, Gao X, Tisdelle L, Eickhoff SB, Liotti M. Naturalizing aesthetics: brain areas for aesthetic appraisal across sensory modalities. Neuroimage. 2011 Sep 1;58(1):250-8. doi: 10.1016/ j.neuroimage.2011.06.012. Epub 2011 Jun 15. PMID: 21699987; PMCID: PMC8005853.

[47] Schlegel A, Alexander P, Fogelson SV, Li X, Lu Z, Kohler PJ, Riley E, Tse PU, Meng M. The artist emerges: visual art learning alters neural structure and function. Neuroimage. 2015 Jan 15;105:440-51. doi:

10.1016/j.neuroimage.2014.11.014. Epub 2014 Nov 15. PMID: 25463452.

[48] Ishizu T, Zeki S. Toward a brain-based theory of beauty. PLoS One. 2011;6(7):e21852. doi: 10.1371/journal.pone.0021852. Epub 2011 Jul 6. PMID: 21755004; PMCID: PMC3130765.

[49] Cattaneo Z, Lega C, Flexas A, Nadal M, Munar E, Cela-Conde CJ. The world can look better: enhancing beauty experience with brain stimulation. Soc Cogn Affect Neurosci. 2014 Nov;9(11):1713-21. doi: 10.1093/scan/nst165. Epub 2013 Oct 15. PMID: 24132459; PMCID: PMC4221210.

[50] Kirk U, Harvey A, Montague PR. Domain expertise insulates against judgment bias by monetary favors through a modulation of ventromedial prefrontal cortex. Proc Natl Acad Sci U S A. 2011 Jun 21;108(25):10332-6. doi: 10.1073/pnas.1019332108. Epub 2011 Jun 6. Erratum in: Proc Natl Acad Sci U S A. 2012 May 1;109(18):7126. PMID: 21646526; PMCID: PMC3121850.

[51] Petrican R, Graham KS, Lawrence AD. Brain-environment alignment during movie watching predicts fluid intelligence and affective function in adulthood. Neuroimage. 2021 Sep;238:118177. doi: 10.1016/j.neuroimage.2021.118177. Epub 2021 May 18. PMID: 34020016; PMCID: PMC8350144.

[52] Lyons KM, Stevenson RA, Owen AM, Stojanoski B. Examining the relationship between measures of autistic traits and neural synchrony during movies in children with and without autism. Neuroimage Clin. 2020;28:102477. doi: 10.1016/j.nicl.2020.102477. Epub 2020 Oct 27. PMID: 33395970; PMCID: PMC7680702.

[53] Bolton TAW, Jochaut D, Giraud AL, Van De Ville D. Brain dynamics in ASD during movie-watching show idiosyncratic functional integration and segregation. Hum Brain Mapp. 2018 Jun;39(6):2391-2404. doi: 10.1002/hbm.24009. Epub 2018 Mar 5. PMID: 29504186; PMCID: PMC5969252.

[54] Mitterschiffthaler MT, Ettinger U, Mehta MA, Mataix-Cols D, Williams SC. Applications of functional magnetic resonance imaging in psychiatry. J Magn Reson Imaging. 2006 Jun;23(6):851-61. doi: 10.1002/jmri.20590. PMID: 16652410.

[55] Garrett AS, Pliszka SR. Neuroimaging of intrinsic connectivity networks: a robust method for assessing functional brain organization

in psychiatric disorders. Braz J Psychiatry. 2020 Jan-Feb;42(1):1-2. doi: 10.1590/1516-4446-2020-0002. PMID: 32022161; PMCID: PMC6986490.

[56] Pearlson GD. Applications of Resting State Functional MR Imaging to Neuropsychiatric Diseases. Neuroimaging Clin N Am. 2017 Nov;27(4):709-723. doi: 10.1016/j.nic.2017.06.005. Epub 2017 Aug 16. PMID: 28985939; PMCID: PMC5743323.

[57] Rikandi E, Pamilo S, Mäntylä T, Suvisaari J, Kieseppä T, Hari R, Seppä M, Raij TT. Precuneus functioning differentiates first-episode psychosis patients during the fantasy movie Alice in Wonderland. Psychol Med. 2017 Feb;47(3):495-506. doi: 10.1017/S00332917 16002609. Epub 2016 Oct 25. PMID: 27776563.

[58] Sung K, Dolcos S, Flor-Henry S, Zhou C, Gasior C, Argo J, Dolcos F. Brain imaging investigation of the neural correlates of observing virtual social interactions. J Vis Exp. 2011 Jul 6;(53):e2379. doi: 10.3791/2379. PMID: 21775952; PMCID: PMC3196171.

[59] Salmi J, Metwaly M, Tohka J, Alho K, Leppämäki S, Tani P, Koski A, Vanderwal T, Laine M. ADHD desynchronizes brain activity during watching a distracted multi-talker conversation. Neuroimage. 2020 Aug 1;216:116352. doi: 10.1016/j.neuroimage.2019.116352. Epub 2019 Nov 12. PMID: 31730921.

[60] Vanderwal T, Eilbott J, Castellanos FX. Movies in the magnet: Naturalistic paradigms in developmental functional neuroimaging. Dev Cogn Neurosci. 2019 Apr;36:100600. doi: 10.1016/ j.dcn.2018.10.004. Epub 2018 Nov 20. PMID: 30551970; PMCID: PMC6969259.

Chapter 5
Integrative Imaging Applications in Attention-Deficit and Hyperactivity Disorder

Abstract

The purposes of this chapter were to investigate further brain structural and functional changes in Attention-deficit and hyperactivity disorder (ADHD) including both combined (AC) and inattention (AI) subtypes compared to typically developed (TD) children with available structural and functional MRI data using multiple advanced imaging methods. For both structural gray matter density (GMD) and interhemispheric correlation, AC group presented significantly larger GMD and VMHC values compared to TD and AI, and relatively close values between AI and TD were found. Specifically, medial orbitofrontal cortex, temporal pole, anterior cingulate, cuneus and supplementary motor area presented both higher values of GDM and VMHC in AC group that might be related to the hyperactivity and attentional deficits in ADHD. Small clusters in the cerebellum, temporal and dorsolateral regions also showed atrophy in AI group compared to TD.

For functional connectivity differences with ICA-DR algorithm, reduced intra- and inter-network connectivities of posterior DMN, visuo-temporal, thalamic-occipital and fronto-temporal networks were observed in AC group compared to TD and AI. However, increased network connectivities in the visual, frontal, anterior DMN, thalamo-temporal and anterior cingulate-FPN regions were found in AC group. Both relative local efficiency and small-worldness weighting factor were lowest in the AC group but highest in the AI group, while the absolute local and global efficiencies were abnormally highest in AC but lowest in AI group. Based on dFNC analysis, reversal dFNC connectogram patterns for most states were revealed in AC compared to TD. The mean dwell time was lower in AC compared to TD, and was significantly lower in the AI patients compared to TD group. Our quantitative multiparametric imaging results showed reliable and rigorous brain changes in ADHD and subtypes compared to TD controls.

Keywords: attention-deficit and hyperactivity disorder, ADHD-inattentive subtype, combined ADHD, typically-developed controls, hyperactivity, attentional deficits, medial orbitofrontal cortex, striatum, insula, cuneus, temporal pole, ventral striatum, hypothalamus, default mode network, frontoparietal network, salience network, motor network, visual network, central executive network, resting state, reversal pattern, functional connectivity, gray matter density, thalamo-cortical network, efficiency, multiparametric imaging, ICA-DR, VMHC, neural correlates, clinical symptom

1. Introduction

1.1. Overview

Attention-deficit and hyperactivity disorder (ADHD) is a relatively high prevalent neurodevelopmental disease, having about 6.3% prevalence rate worldwide based on the Diagnostic and Statistical Manual of mental disorders (DSM-IV) criteria [1, 2]. It had been reported that age and family socioeconomic status affected the prevalence of ADHD in children and adolescents, with more comorbid symptoms such as less impulsivity additionally in adults [1, 3]. ADHD could be classified into the primarily combined ADHD (ADHC-C or AC) and ADHD-inattentive (ADHC-I or AI) subtypes from the typically-developed (TD) controls [4]. Disruptions of brain anatomical and functional networks together with abnormal network topology and connectivity patterns had been reported in ADHD with neuroimaging data recently [3, 5-7]. The purposes of this section are to review the brief findings of ADHD-related imaging studies and subtypes including impairments of attentional/reward/motor networks, and outline the objectives of our comprehensive investigation for this chapter.

For instance, it had been reported that both intra- and inter- network hyper-connectivities were observed in ADHD (especially AC and not AI) group compared to TD, including higher within-anterior DMN, inter- CEN-SN, subcortical-VN and DMN-SN connections in patients compared to TD children [5]. On the other hand, lower large-scale network modularity was also present in AC (not in the AI) subtype in addition to greater loss of network segregation, and was associated with the behavioral and internalization phenotypic scores in these abnormal children. With 8-week brain computer interface-based intervention, the hyper-connectivity between task-positive networks (such as SN, CEN and MN) and task-negative networks (such as anterior DMN) were reduced, with less associated inattentive/internalizing problems through renormalization of functional network processing such as SN [8]. Moreover, the function connectivity of MRI (fcMRI) between DMN and SN correlated with ADHD symptomatic total score, and inter- MN-CEN fcMRI correlated with hyperactivity index in ADHD children while inter- DMN and limbic network impairments were exhibited more in the adult patients [3]. Abnormal structural and functional connectivities of DMN, MN and cerebellum together with deterioration of fronto-striato-thalamic tract in ADHD-C as well as FPN and VN disruption in ADHD-I subtypes were consistently implicated, highlighting network organization differences in two sub-types and from controls [9]. Additionally, ADHD-I patients had higher nodal degree (functional connectivity strength) in the hippocampus compared to both AC and TD groups, also higher in the supramarginal gyrus/calcarine and superior occipital cortex than AC as well as higher amygdala degree than TD. And ADHD-C group had further lower nodal degree in the rolandic operculum and middle temporal pole than TD controls, although higher in the subcortical putamen and anterior cingulate [10]. Lower nodal efficiency and functional connectivities in the DMN and MN in AC compared to TD groups were validated in another study, and correlated with dimensional ADHD clinical scores [11]. Also combinations of fcMRI with ReHo and fALFF utilizing abnormal functional activity and connectivity patterns could reach high classification specificity (85%) for identifying ADHD patients from controls [12]. Classifiers incorporating multiple impaired networks in ADHD such as intra-DMN and inter- SN-DMN/CEN connectivities in both children and adults could reach 84% accuracy of ADHD-healthy controls (HC) classification in children and 81% in adults [12].

Furthermore, the functional dysconnectivities of these specific networks including DMN, FPN, SN and MN (e.g., hyper inter- FPN-DMN and FPN-CEN but hypo FPN-SN and FPN-VN connections) altered attention and sensory functions of multimodal integration as well as high cognitive-level processes such as reward enforcement and response inhibition in ADHD [13, 14]. Further reduced activation in the fronto-striatal regions including multiple frontal clusters, striatal caudate and globus pallidus in response inhibition task were demonstrated in ADHD children, in addition to the less intensity of superior parietal lobe (sensorimotor area) in the selective attention task in ADHD compared to controls [15]. The neural hypofunction in the frontostriatal and FPN circuits were replicated in other response inhibition tasks in ADHD with more recent studies and through utilization of advanced statistical analysis methods [16]. Interestingly, the inattention symptomatic level modulated the fcMRI between DMN and FPN, while the cortico-subcortical networks such as SN determined the reward processing in ADHD [17]. The reinforcement such as monetary incentive delayed task improved reward responsiveness that was selectively associated with SN in ADHD patients, together with compensatory visual network [18]. Lower intra-sensory as well as inter- sensory and DMN stepwise functional connectivities were identified, and were inversely correlated with the ADHD clinical severity scale [19]. In addition to the conventional fcMRI, novel dynamic functional network correlation (dFNC) revealed disrupted dynamics such as more dwell time in the hyper-connected states but less in the segregated network states in ADHD [20]. Also connectomics method with maturational lag analysis observed significant dynamic correlation differences between DMN and FPN/SN (two task-positive networks), that might underlie the pathophysiology of attentional dysfunction in ADHD [21].

1.2. Objectives

Brain functional connectivity and activity changes had been reported in ADHD and subtypes, especially inter- and intra-network modulations. The purposes of this chapter are to investigate further brain structural and functional changes in ADHD combined and inattention subtypes compared to typically developed children with available structural and functional MRI data using multiple advanced imaging methods. ICA-DR and dFNC were further implemented in addition to conventional VBM/VMHC analyses with the hope to reveal the underlying disease mechanism of ADHD and provide therapeutic guidance with thorough detailed review and discussion.

2. Methods

2.1. Participants

From a large cohort of ADHD-200 samples (http://fcon_1000. projects.nitrc.org/indi/adhd200/index.html), 25 TD children, 7 ADHD-AC and 9 ADHD-AI child patients were selected to study ADHD-related brain changes from TD and subtype differentiation including AI. Imaging data were downloaded after approval from the website managed at NITRC and provided by the Peking

University in Beijing, China. More information was available at the INDI Prospective Data Sharing Samples ADHD project hosted by NITRC [22-25].

The participants were recruited for MRI scans with clinical diagnosis such as the ADHD Rating Scale (ADHD-RS) IV for measuring ADHD dimensional symptoms, and participants also met the following criteria: right-handedness and full scale Wechsler Intelligence Scale for Chinese Children-Revised (WISCC-R) score of greater than 80, no lifetime history of head trauma with loss of consciousness, no history of neurological disease and no diagnosis of either schizophrenia, affective disorder, pervasive development disorder or substance abuse. Psychostimulant medications were withheld at least 48 hours prior to scanning, and study was approved by the Research Ethics Review Board at Institute of Mental Health of the Peking University [26-29].

2.2. Imaging Parameters and Data Processing

MRI experiments were performed using the 3T scanner with standardized imaging protocols. The 3D MPRAGE sequence was run with TR/TI/TE=2530/1100/3.39 ms, flip angle=9°, matrix size=256 x 208 x 176, resolution=1 x 1x 1 mm³ for reference image used in RS-fMRI activity/connectivity/conductivity maps, as well as for structural voxel-based morphometry (VBM) analysis. For the resting-state (RS)-fMRI data acquired under relaxing condition, a standard gradient-echo EPI sequence (TR/TE=2000/30 msec, flip angle=90°, number of volumes=236, spatial resolution=3.13 x 3.13 x 3.6 mm³) was utilized.

The MRI and fMRI images were processed with in-house developed scripts to derive the VMHC, VBM, ICA-DR, resting-state functional connectivity (RSFC) and fractional ALFF (fALFF) maps, as described in details in previous chapters and our recent works [30-32]. Between-group comparisons of quantitative post-processed images were performed with advanced statistical tools using AFNI package and FMRIB Software Library (FSL, http://www.fmrib.ox.ac.uk/fsl) toolbox. Graph theory based small-worldness systematic analysis was computed to the functional connectivity of MRI (fcMRI) data with correlation matrix generated from 116 seeds-based resting state functional connectivity (RSFC), and comparisons between patients and controls were performed.

Relatively new dynamic dFNC connectogram and regional homogeneity (ReHo) map together with typical VMHC, ICA-DR, fALFF, and small-worldness analyses were performed to the data cohorts. Six typical and important functional networks were used for dFNC analysis as in previous chapter, including default mode network (DMN), frontoparietal network (FPN), salience network (SN), motor network (MN), visual network (VN) and central executive network (CEN or EN). In addition, regional homogeneity (ReHo) map was generated to reflect spatially local synchrony of spontaneous neuronal activities, after preprocessing the fMRI data such as motion correction and low-pass filtering using Analysis of Functional NeuroImages (AFNI, http://afni.nimh.nih.gov) 3dReHo command. The coefficient of concordance between time series of center and neighborhood voxels was computed (e.g., 27 voxels were used as default values including the face, edge and node-wise spatial neighbors) for each voxel of the 4D fMRI data, and Z-score was derived for voxel-wise between-group comparison and global mean statistical quantification [33-35].

3. Results

Significant gray matter density differences among three groups using VBM with $P<0.01$ were displayed in Figure 1. Comparing

ADHD-C group to TD participants, higher gray matter densities were observed in the medial orbitofrontal cortex, anterior cingulate, DMN including posterior cingulate and medial prefrontal cortex (MPFC), cuneus, superior temporal region and small clusters in the supplementary motor area in AC group (Figure 1A). Comparing AC to AI groups, higher gray matter densities with similar pattern as in A with less significant level was present, together with additional somatosensory and motor areas in AC (Figure 1B). Gray matter atrophies in the subcortical caudate/putamen, amygdala and cerebellum were identified in AC group compared to AI on the other hand. Small clusters in the cerebellum, temporal and caudate regions also showed higher GMD in AI group compared to TD (Figure 1C), but atrophies in scattered visual, insular and motor areas.

Figure 2 demonstrated VMHC differences among three groups (P<0.001). Higher interhemispheric correlations were identified in large areas of occipital cortex, cerebellum and thalamus, scattered regions of anterior temporal, striatum, basal ganglia, amygdala, cuneus, orbitofrontal, anterior cingulate and supplementary motor areas for the AC group compared to TD participants. Slightly lower VMHC in the cuneus was found in AC group as well. Comparing AC to AI group, similar difference pattern was identified, including higher VMHC in the occipital, temporal, insula, anterior cingulate and orbitofrontal regions in AC. Small clusters in the rectus, amygdala, hippocampus and supplementary motor area showed higher VMHC in AI group compared to TD, but VMHC was lower in the superior temporal and lingual regions in the AI group.

ICA-DR algorithm identified intra- and inter-network connectivity differences comparing AC to TD groups (Figure 3, P<0.01). For instance, lower visuo-temporal, posterior DMN, thalamic-occipital, FPN-VN and fronto-temporal network connectivities were observed in AC group compared to TD. On the other hand, increased intra-

and inter- visual, thalamo-temporal, visuomotor, CEN-DMN, frontal, temporal and FPN-CEN connectivities were also present in AC group, possibly for compensation and re-routing. Figure 4 showed the ICA-DR based intra- and inter-network connectivity differences comparing AC to AI groups (P<0.01) with some common network changes as in Figure 3 with slight differences. Lower VN-SN, VN-MN, thalamic-occipital, frontal-DMN, SN-temporal and fronto-temporal inter-network connectivities were observed in AC group compared to AI. However, increased intra- and inter- visual, frontal, thalamo-temporal, VN-DMN, CEN-SN, SN-FPN, frontal-SN, temporo-occipital and CEN-FPN network connectivities were also present in AC group.

Small clusters in the insula, posterior cingulate and somatosensory cortices showed lower connectivities in AI compared to TD groups, but higher in small inferior parietal region, cerebellum, caudate and MPFC (Figure 5, P<0.01). Small-worldness analysis with the functional connectivity data identified lowest relative local efficiency and small-worldness configuration factor in AC group, but highest in the AI group. Similar global efficiencies were present in three groups, with lowest absolute local efficiency in AI but highest in AC groups (Figure 6).

Frequency and mean dwell time of all 6 six states were demonstrated in Figure 7 (A&C for ADHD-AC subtype B&D for AI respectively). Compared to AI group, AC group tended to stay in lower dwell time states more often, presenting a less optimal distribution of brain dynamic states. The mean dwell time was lower in AI and AC patients compared to TD group, with significant differences between AI and TD (P=0.025) and a trend (P=0.07) in AC compared to TD groups (Figure 8A). However, no significant differences of fractional occupancy between groups existed (Figure 8B). Connectogram of six states in TD children and ADHD-AC group were displayed in Figure 9 A and B respectively. Reversal dFNC pattern in AC for most states (S1-6 except state 4) was revealed compared to TD. Group mean functional fALFF and ReHo images presented no significant statistical differences among three groups. Slightly lower frontal neural activity but higher in the cerebellum of ADHD-C compared to TD were identified (Figure 10). On the other hand, higher synchrony in the motor and visual areas primarily but lower subcortical putamen and cerebellum ReHo in AC were revealed as well.

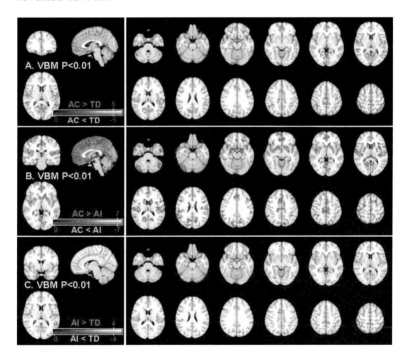

Figure 1. *Significant gray matter density differences among three groups using VBM with P<0.01. A: Comparing ADHD-C (AC) group to TD participants: higher gray matter densities (GMD) were observed in the medial orbitofrontal cortex, anterior cingulate, posterior cingulate, cuneus, superior temporal region and small clusters in the supplementary motor area in AC group (red color). B: Comparing AC to AI groups, higher GMD with similar pattern as in A were present, together with additional somatosensory areas and motor areas. Gray*

matter atrophies in the subcortical caudate/putamen, amygdala and cerebellum were identified in AC group on the other hand (blue). C: Small clusters in the cerebellum, temporal, caudate regions also showed higher GMD in AI group compared to TD, but atrophies in scattered regions of the visual, insular and motor areas existed for AI as well.

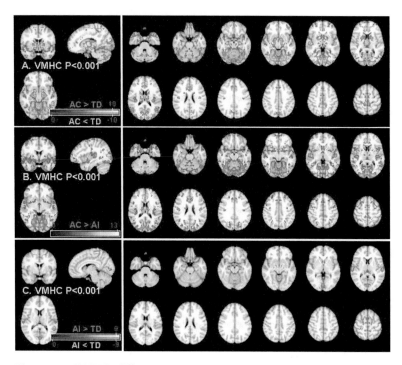

Figure 2. *VMHC differences among three groups (P<0.001). A: Higher interhemispheric correlations were identified in large areas of occipital cortex, cerebellum and thalamus, scattered regions of anterior temporal, striatum, basal ganglia, amygdala, cuneus, orbitofrontal, anterior cingulate and supplementary motor areas for the AC group compared to TD participants. Slightly lower VMHC in the cuneus were found in AD group as well. B: Comparing AC to AI group, similar pattern as in A were found in AC group, including higher VMHC in the occipital, temporal, insula, anterior cingulate and orbitofrontal regions. C: Small clusters in the rectus, amygdala, hippocampus and supplementary motor area showed higher VMHC in AI group compared to TD, but VMHC were lower in the superior temporal and lingual regions in the AI group.*

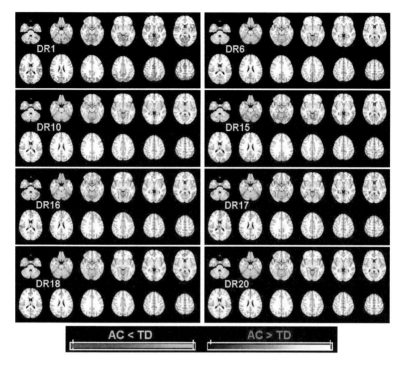

Figure 3. *ICA-DR algorithm identified intra- and inter-network connectivity differences comparing AC to TD groups (P<0.01). Lower visuo-temporal, posterior DMN, thalamic-occipital, temporal-SN, VN-FPN and occipito-frontal network connectivities were observed in AC group compared to TD (blue color). On the other hand, increased intra- and inter- visual, thalamo-temporal, visuomotor, VN-DMN, CEN-SN, FPN-CEN connectivities were also present in AC group (red color), possibly for compensation and normal regulation.*

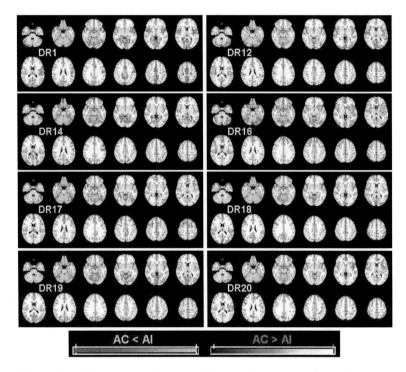

Figure 4. *ICA-DR based intra- and inter-network connectivity differences comparing AC to AI groups (P<0.01) identified some common network changes as in Figure 3 with sight differences. Lower VN-SN, VN-MN, thalamic-occipital, frontal-DMN, SN-temporal and fronto-temporal inter-network connectivities were observed in AC group compared to AI (blue color). However, increased intra- and inter- visual, frontal, thalamo-temporal, VN-DMN, CEN-SN, SN-FPN, temporo-occipital and FPN-CEN network connectivities were also present in AC group (red color), similarly as in Figure 3.*

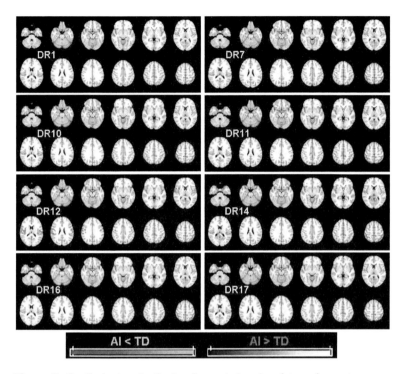

Figure 5. *Small clusters in the insula, posterior cingulate and somatosensory showed lower connectivities in AI compared to TD groups, but higher in small inferior parietal, cerebellum, caudate and medial frontal regions (P<0.01).*

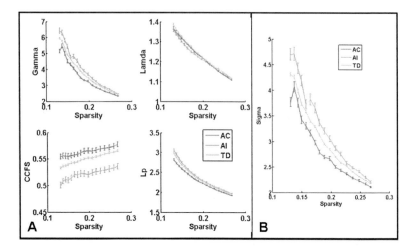

Figure 6. *Small-worldness analysis with the functional connectivity data presented lowest relative local efficiency and small-worldness configuration factor in AC group, but highest in the AI group. Similar global efficiencies were present in three groups, with lowest absolute local and global efficiencies in AI but highest in AC groups.*

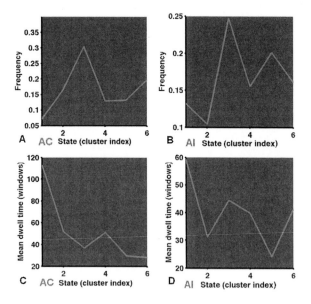

Figure 7. *Frequency and mean dwell time of all 6 six states in ADHD-C (A&C) and ADHD-I (AI, B&D). Compared to AI group, AC group tended to stay in lower dwell time states more often, with a less optimal distribution of brain dynamic states.*

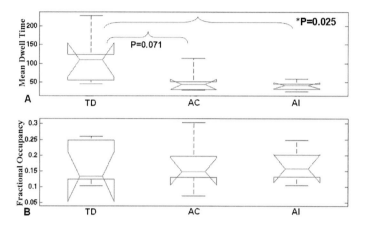

Figure 8. *A: The mean dwell time was lower in AI & AC patients compared to TD group, with significant differences between AI and TD (P=0.025) and a trend (P=0.07) in AC compared to TD groups. B: No significant differences of fractional occupancy between groups.*

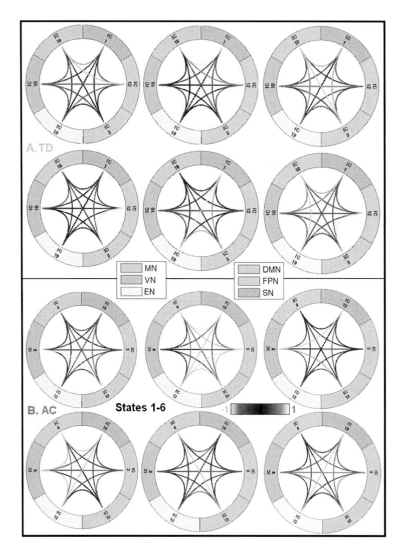

Figure 9. *Connectogram of six states in TD children (A) and ADHD-AC group (B). Reversal dFNC patterns of majorities of inter-network connections in AC for most states (S1-S6 except S4) such as S1 and S5 listed as in the left-most and middle-bottom panels were revealed compared to TD group.*

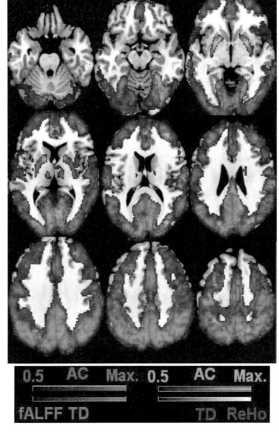

Figure 10. *Group mean functional fALFF and ReHo images without significant statistical differences. Slightly lower frontal neural activity (red in AC vs. violet color in TD) but higher in the cerebellum in ADHD-AC compared to TD were identified. On the other hand, higher synchrony in the motor and visual areas primarily but lower subcortical putamen and cerebellum ReHo in AC were revealed as well (green in AC vs. gold color in TD groups).*

4. Summary and Discussion

4.1. Summary of Results

For both structural gray matter density (GMD) and interhemispheric correlation, ADHD-AC group presented significantly larger GMD (such as in DMN and MN) and VMHC (such as in occipital/thalamus/cerebellum) values compared to TD and AI, and relatively close values between AI and TD were observed additionally. For instance, medial orbitofrontal cortex, temporal pole, anterior cingulate cortex, cuneus and supplementary motor area presented both higher values of GDM and VMHC in AC group that might be related to the hyperactivity and attentional deficits. Small clusters in the cerebellum, temporal and dorsolateral regions also showed atrophy in AI group compared to TD. And extra-large areas in the occipital lobe, cerebellum and thalamus also presented higher VMHC in AC compared to AI and AD groups. Moreover, small clusters in the rectus, amygdala, hippocampus and supplementary motor area showed higher gray matter density in AI group compared to TD.

For functional connectivity differences with ICA-DR algorithm, reduced intra- and inter-network connectivities of VN-SN, thalamic-occipital, MN-VN and CEN-SN networks were observed in AC group compared to TD and AI. However, increased intra- and inter-network connectivities of the VN, anterior DMN, oribitofrontal, thalamo-temporal, and CEN-FPN regions were found in AC group. Consistent with reported findings, affected typical networks of DMN, CEN, FPN, SN, MN, VN connections implicated disruption of internalized cognitive state integration, motivation, motor, visuospatial ability, executive control and inhibitory functions. Small clusters in the posterior cingulate and somatosensory cortices showed lower connectivities in AI compared to TD groups, but higher in small regions of cerebellum, caudate, inferior parietal and medial frontal cortices. Both relative local efficiency and small-worldness weighting factor were lowest in the AC group, but highest in the AI group, while the absolute local and global efficiencies were abnormally highest in AC but lowest in AI group. The higher efficiency values in AI group might indicate the intermediate stage and possible protective mechanism in patients. Based on dFNC analysis, reversal dFNC connectogram patterns in AC compared to TD for most states (five out of all six) were revealed. Similar to the epilepsy patient results [35], AC group tended to stay in lower dwell time states more often, with a less optimal distribution of brain dynamic states. The mean dwell time was lower in AC compared to TD, and reached significance in the AI patients in comparison to TD group. Taken together, our multiparametric functional connectivity/activity results were consistent with the typical imaging deficits in ADHD, with additional dynamic connectogram and high-level inter-network modulation as well as conductivity/structural abnormality confirmations.

4.2. Comparison with Previous Multimodal Findings

Lower white matter fractional anisotropy (FA) values were observed in the corona radiata, longitudinal fasciculus, thalamic radiation, internal capsule and the sagittal striatum in adults with childhood ADHD [36]. Increased axial but decreased radial diffusivity values as an indicator of demyelination were also found in the posterior cingulum bundle for the children and adolescents with ADHD compared to controls. And increased FA in the cingulum was related to the executive function score [37]. FA of the superior longitudinal fasciculus was correlated with the ADHD symptoms, while the inferior fronto-occipital fasciculus FA together with the attentional network fcMRI correlated with the phenotypic and genetic data [38]. Out of the multi-modal imaging features including gray matter volume/thickness and functional/structural connectivities as well as global small-worldness topological quantifications, inferior frontal gyrus (IFG) nodal efficiency, MFC-inferior parietal lobe (IPL) fcMRI and amygdala volume (all on the right side) contributed significantly to the differentiation between ADHD probands and controls with a relatively high accuracy of 0.9 [39]. In addition, higher MPFC nodal efficiency was associated with the inattentive and hyperactive/impulsive remission symptom, while higher MFC-IPL fcMRI was linked to symptom persistence in adults with childhood ADHD. Two distinct white matter functional network patterns in ADHD were identified; namely, the hyperactivity-related hot network such as DMN and MN as well as the inattention-related cold network including attentional networks such as SN and CEN [40]. Furthermore, multimodal deficits in both networks were related to more symptoms in ADHD and gray matter atrophy corresponded to the abnormal white matter indices in the prefrontal cortex [41].

4.3 Neural correlates of ADHD Clinical Symptoms

For functional connectivity metric, the abnormal and atypical values of connections between sensorimotor and basal ganglia/cerebellum/anterior cingulate cortex (ACC)/supplementary motor area (SMA) were associated with motor function and visuospatial processing deficits in ADHD with developmental coordination disorder [42]. Furthermore, age-related aberrant brain network changes in the IFG/insula and middle temporal gyrus (MTL) were related to the cognitive function deficits in ADHD [43]. And less neural activity in the ACC and IFG was associated with poorer rapid visual processing test while activation in the superior parietal lobule was associated with pattern recognition and memory correct response percentage in ADHD youths using the counting Stroop task fMRI paradigm [44]. In addition, functional activities in the sensory network and DMN were correlated to the ADHD symptom such as inattention and hyperactivity burden that had distinct pattern across the executive function domains [45].

For gray matter volumetry, cortical atrophy in the superior temporal gyrus (STG) and ACC on the left side was identified in ADHD children, and STG volume correlated with working memory tests [46]. Also gray matter atrophy in the frontal/parietal/temporal lobes together with larger volume in the calcarine and occipitotemporal region were found to be related to the worse symptom severity [47]. The IFG and insular/superior frontal gray matter reduction were associated with working memory and inattention, suggesting important role of these regions in ADHD remission across adolescence and adulthood [48]. And gray matter global network organization was altered with higher local subcortical nodal degree such as in the amygdala but lower in the cortical regions including ACC/posterior cingulate cortex (PCC) and MTL, indicating loss of inhibitory and regulation abilities in ADHD [49]. Moreover, higher intra-class correlation of PCC and ventral precuneus were likely to reflect underlying the pathophysiology and heterogeneity of ADHD [50]. Finally, gray matter atrophy and white matter dysconnectivity in frontal regions and functional disconnection in the DMN and FPN patterns co-occurred in ADHD children, while reduced fronto-striatal gray matter volume and disrupted inter-connected white matter integrity consolidated the robust imaging findings [47, 51].

4.4 Therapeutic Effects in ADHD

After the brain-computer-interface (CBI) training, degree centrality and clustering coefficient in brain networks such as SN and DMN were reduced and linked to less inattentive/internalizing problems with more random and renormalized network reconfiguration in ADHD children [52]. With the deep transcranial magnetic stimulation (tTMS) treatment, increased activations in the DLPFC, parietal cortex and insula/IFG during working-memory tests were detected that also correlated with inattention/memory symptom improvements [53]. Furthermore, treated participants showed less brain structural changes of volume reductions in the basal ganglia, ACC and amygdala from child to adulthood compared to non-treated populations [54]. Alternative treatment of Chinese medicine, Baicalin (Huanqin, Scutellaria) significantly increased dopamine abundance level in the striatum compared to saline sham treatment, and similarly for the conventional methylphenidate that increased dopamine in both DLPFC and striatum regions [55]. And both medicine demonstrated therapeutic effects of lower hyperactivity and less spatial learning and memory deficits in treated patients. Some tailored clinical interventions for ADHD had been tested including the neuro-stimulation therapy that could enhance key network response to rectify individual brain dynamics with better clinical symptom such as more stable emotion based on the whole-brain connectome model [56]. Further genetic factors had also been investigated; for instance, lower local gyrification index scores were found in the ADHD with prenatal alcohol exposure in several brain regions including prefrontal, insula, cingulate, temporal and parietal cortices, and correlated with the worse clinical-behavioral performance such as lower intelligence test, higher hyperactivity/impulsivity and poor behavioral regulation scores [57]. Integration of cell and animal model, bioinformatics, genetics and multimodal imaging to explore biological and multiomics pathways for correcting ADHD were proposed and could interact with the brain structural and functional changes to reveal the underlying biological complexity and disease mechanism [58, 59]. Multi-center trials with vitamin A and D supplementation on ADHD children treatment, long-acting combination therapy together with some optimal patient and caregiver management tools such as telehealth service model for reducing distress had also been evaluated and implemented for better therapeutic outcome [60-62].

4.5. Conclusion

Consistent gray matter density and interhemispheric correlation deficits were observed in ADHD-Combined type compared to AI and TD groups, with abnormally higher values in the DMN, medial orbitofrontal cortex, temporal pole, anterior cingulate, cuneus and supplementary motor areas. Furthermore, reduced intra- and inter-network connectivities of VN-SN, VN-FPN, DMN-VN, thalamic-occipital and fronto-temporal networks were observed in AC group compared to TD and AI, in addition to the increased inter-network connectivities of visual, anterior DMN, frontal-SN including orbitofrontal and CEN, thalamo-temporal and CEN-FPN. Both relative local efficiency and small-worldness weighting factor were lowest in the AC group but highest in the AI group, while the absolute local and global efficiencies were abnormally highest in AC but lowest in AI group. The higher efficiency values in AI group might indicate the intermediate stage and possible protective mechanism in patients. Reversal dFNC connectogram patterns in AC compared to TD for most states were revealed. Also similar to the epilepsy patients results in our previous work [35] and consistent with the relatively high comorbidity (~30-40%) of ADHD in epilepsy for children [63], AC group tended to stay in lower dwell time states more often with a less optimal distribution of brain dynamic states. Our quantitative multiparametric imaging results showed reliable and rigorous brain changes such as reduced connectivity pattern of task positive networks including CEN, SN and FPN in addition to abnormally higher inter- DMN-CEN and DMN-SN connections together with attentional/memory and inhibitory functional deficits in ADHD and subtypes compared to TD group.

References

[1] Rockhill CM, Carlisle LL, Qu P, Vander Stoep A, French W, Zhou C, Myers K. Primary Care Management of Children with Attention-Deficit/Hyperactivity Disorder Appears More Assertive Following Brief Psychiatric Intervention Compared with Single Session Consultation. J Child Adolesc Psychopharmacol. 2020 Jun;30(5):285-292. doi: 10.1089/cap.2020.0013. Epub 2020 Mar 11. PMID: 32167784; PMCID: PMC7310318.

[2] American Psychiatric Association (2013). Diagnostic and Statistical Manual of Mental Disorders (5th ed.). Arlington: American Psychiatric Publishing. pp. 59–65. ISBN 978-0-89042-555-8.

[3] Guo X, Yao D, Cao Q, Liu L, Zhao Q, Li H, Huang F, Wang Y, Qian Q, Wang Y, Calhoun VD, Johnstone SJ, Sui J, Sun L. Shared and distinct resting functional connectivity in children and adults with attention-deficit/hyperactivity disorder. Transl Psychiatry. 2020 Feb 12;10(1):65. doi: 10.1038/s41398-020-0740-y. PMID: 32066697; PMCID: PMC7026417.

[4] Brown MR, Sidhu GS, Greiner R, Asgarian N, Bastani M, Silverstone PH, Greenshaw AJ, Dursun SM. ADHD-200 Global Competition: diagnosing ADHD using personal characteristic data can outperform resting state fMRI measurements. Front Syst Neurosci. 2012 Sep 28;6:69. doi: 10.3389/fnsys.2012.00069. PMID: 23060754; PMCID: PMC3460316.

[5] Qian X, Castellanos FX, Uddin LQ, Loo BRY, Liu S, Koh HL, Poh XWW, Fung D, Guan C, Lee TS, Lim CG, Zhou J. Large-scale brain functional network topology disruptions underlie symptom heterogeneity in children with attention-deficit/hyperactivity disorder. Neuroimage Clin. 2019;21:101600. doi: 10.1016/j.nicl.2018.11.010. Epub 2018 Nov 19. PMID: 30472167; PMCID: PMC6411599.

[6] Bush G. Cingulate, frontal, and parietal cortical dysfunction in attention-deficit/hyperactivity disorder. Biol Psychiatry. 2011 Jun 15;69(12):1160-7. doi: 10.1016/j.biopsych.2011.01.022. Epub 2011 Apr 13. PMID: 21489409; PMCID: PMC3109164.

[7] Posner J, Park C, Wang Z. Connecting the dots: a review of resting connectivity MRI studies in attention-deficit/hyperactivity disorder. Neuropsychol Rev. 2014 Mar;24(1):3-15. doi: 10.1007/s11065-014-9251-z. Epub 2014 Feb 5. PMID: 24496902; PMCID: PMC4119002.

[8] Qian X, Loo BRY, Castellanos FX, Liu S, Koh HL, Poh XWW, Krishnan R, Fung D, Chee MW, Guan C, Lee TS, Lim CG, Zhou J. Brain-computer-interface-based intervention re-normalizes brain functional network topology in children with attention deficit/hyperactivity disorder. Transl Psychiatry. 2018 Aug 10;8(1):149. doi: 10.1038/s41398-018-0213-8. PMID: 30097579; PMCID: PMC6086861.

[9] Saad JF, Griffiths KR, Korgaonkar MS. A Systematic Review of Imaging Studies in the Combined and Inattentive Subtypes of Attention Deficit Hyperactivity Disorder. Front Integr Neurosci. 2020 Jun 24;14:31. doi: 10.3389/fnint.2020.00031. PMID: 32670028; PMCID: PMC7327109.

[10] Saad JF, Griffiths KR, Kohn MR, Clarke S, Williams LM, Korgaonkar MS. Regional brain network organization distinguishes the combined and inattentive subtypes of Attention Deficit Hyperactivity Disorder. Neuroimage Clin. 2017 May 22;15:383-390. doi: 10.1016/j.nicl.2017.05.016. PMID: 28580295; PMCID: PMC5447655.

[11] Wang M, Hu Z, Liu L, Li H, Qian Q, Niu H. Disrupted functional brain connectivity networks in children with attention-deficit/hyperactivity disorder: evidence from resting-state functional near-infrared spectroscopy. Neurophotonics. 2020 Jan;7(1):015012. doi: 10.1117/1.NPh.7.1.015012. Epub 2020 Mar 11. PMID: 32206679; PMCID: PMC7064804.

[12] Cheng W, Ji X, Zhang J, Feng J. Individual classification of ADHD patients by integrating multiscale neuroimaging markers and advanced pattern recognition techniques. Front Syst Neurosci. 2012 Aug 6;6:58. doi: 10.3389/fnsys.2012.00058. PMID: 22888314; PMCID: PMC3412279.

[13] Gao Y, Shuai D, Bu X, Hu X, Tang S, Zhang L, Li H, Hu X, Lu L, Gong Q, Huang X. Impairments of large-scale functional networks in attention-deficit/hyperactivity disorder: a meta-analysis of resting-state functional connectivity. Psychol Med. 2019 Nov;49(15):2475-2485. doi: 10.1017/S003329171900237X. Epub 2019 Sep 10. PMID: 31500674.

[14] Sripada C, Kessler D, Fang Y, Welsh RC, Prem Kumar K, Angstadt M. Disrupted network architecture of the resting brain in attention-deficit/hyperactivity disorder. Hum Brain Mapp. 2014 Sep;35(9): 4693-705. doi: 10.1002/hbm.22504. Epub 2014 Mar 25. PMID: 24668728; PMCID: PMC6869736.

[15] Booth JR, Burman DD, Meyer JR, Lei Z, Trommer BL, Davenport ND, Li W, Parrish TB, Gitelman DR, Mesulam MM. Larger deficits in brain networks for response inhibition than for visual selective attention in attention deficit hyperactivity disorder (ADHD). J Child Psychol Psychiatry. 2005 Jan;46(1):94-111. doi: 10.1111/j.1469-7610.2004.00337.x. PMID: 15660647.

[16] Dickstein SG, Bannon K, Castellanos FX, Milham MP. The neural correlates of attention deficit hyperactivity disorder: an ALE meta-analysis. J Child Psychol Psychiatry. 2006 Oct;47(10):1051-62. doi: 10.1111/j.1469-7610.2006.01671.x. PMID: 17073984.

[17] Oldehinkel M, Beckmann CF, Franke B, Hartman CA, Hoekstra PJ, Oosterlaan J, Heslenfeld D, Buitelaar JK, Mennes M. Functional connectivity in cortico-subcortical brain networks underlying reward processing in attention-deficit/hyperactivity disorder. Neuroimage Clin. 2016 Oct 8;12:796-805. doi: 10.1016/j.nicl.2016.10.006. PMID: 27818941; PMCID: PMC5081416.

[18] Valmiki M, Fawzy P, Valmiki S, Aid MA, Chaitou AR, Zahid M, Khan S. Reinforcement and Compensatory Mechanisms in Attention-Deficit Hyperactivity Disorder: A Systematic Review of Case-Control Studies. Cureus. 2021 Mar 5;13(3):e13718. doi: 10.7759/cureus.13718. PMID: 33833929; PMCID: PMC8018873.

[19] Pretus C, Marcos-Vidal L, Martínez-García M, Picado M, Ramos-Quiroga JA, Richarte V, Castellanos FX, Sepulcre J, Desco M, Vilarroya Ó, Carmona S. Stepwise functional connectivity reveals altered sensory-multimodal integration in medication-naïve adults with attention deficit hyperactivity disorder. Hum Brain Mapp. 2019 Nov 1;40(16):4645-4656. doi: 10.1002/hbm.24727. Epub 2019 Jul 19. PMID: 31322305; PMCID: PMC6865796.

[20] Shappell HM, Duffy KA, Rosch KS, Pekar JJ, Mostofsky SH, Lindquist MA, Cohen JR. Children with attention-deficit/hyperactivity disorder spend more time in hyperconnected network states and less time in segregated network states as revealed by dynamic connectivity analysis. Neuroimage. 2021 Apr 1;229:117753. doi: 10.1016/j.neuroimage.2021.117753. Epub 2021 Jan 14. PMID: 33454408; PMCID: PMC7979530.

[21] Sripada CS, Kessler D, Angstadt M. Lag in maturation of the brain's intrinsic functional architecture in attention-deficit/hyperactivity

disorder. Proc Natl Acad Sci U S A. 2014 Sep 30;111(39):14259-64. doi: 10.1073/pnas.1407787111. Epub 2014 Sep 15. PMID: 25225387; PMCID: PMC4191792.

[22] McLeod KR, Langevin LM, Dewey D, Goodyear BG. Atypical within- and between-hemisphere motor network functional connections in children with developmental coordination disorder and attention-deficit/hyperactivity disorder. Neuroimage Clin. 2016 Jun 28;12:157-64. doi: 10.1016/j.nicl.2016.06.019. PMID: 27419066; PMCID: PMC4936600.

[23] Zhu CZ, Zang YF, Cao QJ, Yan CG, He Y, Jiang TZ, Sui MQ, Wang YF. Fisher discriminative analysis of resting-state brain function for attention-deficit/hyperactivity disorder. Neuroimage. 2008 Mar 1;40(1):110-20. doi: 10.1016/j.neuroimage.2007.11.029. Epub 2007 Dec 3. PMID: 18191584.

[24] Zang YF, He Y, Zhu CZ, Cao QJ, Sui MQ, Liang M, Tian LX, Jiang TZ, Wang YF. Altered baseline brain activity in children with ADHD revealed by resting-state functional MRI. Brain Dev. 2007 Mar;29(2):83-91. doi: 10.1016/j.braindev.2006.07.002. Epub 2006 Aug 17. Erratum in: Brain Dev. 2012 Apr;34(4):336. PMID: 16919409.

[25] Wang L, Zhu C, He Y, Zang Y, Cao Q, Zhang H, Zhong Q, Wang Y. Altered small-world brain functional networks in children with attention-deficit/hyperactivity disorder. Hum Brain Mapp. 2009 Feb;30(2):638-49. doi: 10.1002/hbm.20530. PMID: 18219621; PMCID: PMC6870909.

[26] Cao Q, Zang Y, Sun L, Sui M, Long X, Zou Q, Wang Y. Abnormal neural activity in children with attention deficit hyperactivity disorder: a resting-state functional magnetic resonance imaging study. Neuroreport. 2006 Jul 17;17(10):1033-6. doi: 10.1097/01.wnr. 0000224769.92454.5d. PMID: 16791098.

[27] Zhao Y, Cui D, Lu W, Li H, Zhang H, Qiu J. Aberrant gray matter volumes and functional connectivity in adolescent patients with ADHD. J Magn Reson Imaging. 2020 Mar;51(3):719-726. doi: 10.1002/jmri.26854. Epub 2019 Jul 2. PMID: 31265198.

[28] Cao X, Cao Q, Long X, Sun L, Sui M, Zhu C, Zuo X, Zang Y, Wang Y. Abnormal resting-state functional connectivity patterns of the putamen in medication-naïve children with attention deficit hyperactivity disorder. Brain Res. 2009 Dec 15;1303:195-206. doi: 10.1016/j.brainres.2009.08.029. Epub 2009 Aug 20. PMID: 19699190.

[29] Tian L, Jiang T, Wang Y, Zang Y, He Y, Liang M, Sui M, Cao Q, Hu S, Peng M, Zhuo Y. Altered resting-state functional connectivity patterns of anterior cingulate cortex in adolescents with attention deficit hyperactivity disorder. Neurosci Lett. 2006 May 29;400(1-2):39-43. doi: 10.1016/j.neulet.2006.02.022. Epub 2006 Feb 28. PMID: 16510242.

[30] Zhou Y. *Functional Neuroimaging with Multiple Modalities: Principle, Device and Applications.* Nova Science Publishers. 2016.

[31] Zhou Y. *Functional Neuroimaging Methods and Frontiers.* Nova Science Publishers. 2018.

[32] Zhou Y. *Multiparametric Imaging in Neurodegenerative Disease.* Nova Science Publishers. 2019.

[33] Zhou Y. *Joint Imaging Applications in General Neurodegenerative Disease: Parkinson's, Frontotemporal, Vascular Dementia and Autism.* Nova Science Publishers. 2021.

[34] Zhou Y. *Imaging and Multiomic Biomarker Applications: Advances in Early Alzheimer's Disease.* Nova Science Publishers. 2020.

[35] Zhou Y. *Typical Imaging in Atypical Parkinson's, Schizophrenia, Epilepsy and Asymptomatic Alzheimer's Disease.* Nova Science Publishers. 2021.

[36] Cortese S, Imperati D, Zhou J, Proal E, Klein RG, Mannuzza S, Ramos-Olazagasti MA, Milham MP, Kelly C, Castellanos FX. White matter alterations at 33-year follow-up in adults with childhood attention-deficit/hyperactivity disorder. Biol Psychiatry. 2013 Oct 15;74(8):591-8. doi: 10.1016/j.biopsych.2013.02.025. Epub 2013 Apr 6. PMID: 23566821;PMCID: PMC3720804.

[37] Chen L, Huang X, Lei D, He N, Hu X, Chen Y, Li Y, Zhou J, Guo L, Kemp GJ, Gong QY. Microstructural abnormalities of the brain white matter in attention-deficit/hyperactivity disorder. J Psychiatry Neurosci. 2015 Jul;40(4):280-7. doi: 10.1503/jpn.140199. PMID: 25853285; PMCID: PMC4478061.

[38] Sudre G, Choudhuri S, Szekely E, Bonner T, Goduni E, Sharp W, Shaw P. Estimating the Heritability of Structural and Functional Brain Connectivity in Families Affected by Attention-Deficit/Hyperactivity Disorder. JAMA Psychiatry. 2017 Jan 1;74(1):76-84. doi: 10.1001/jamapsychiatry.2016.3072. PMID: 27851842; PMCID: PMC7418037.

[39] Luo Y, Alvarez TL, Halperin JM, Li X. Multimodal neuroimaging-based prediction of adult outcomes in childhood-onset ADHD using

ensemble learning techniques. Neuroimage Clin. 2020;26:102238. doi: 10.1016/j.nicl. 2020.102238. Epub 2020 Mar 7. PMID: 32182578; PMCID: PMC7076568.

[40] Bu X, Liang K, Lin Q, Gao Y, Qian A, Chen H, Chen W, Wang M, Yang C, Huang X. Exploring white matter functional networks in children with attention-deficit/hyperactivity disorder. Brain Commun. 2020 Jul 21;2(2):fcaa113. doi: 10.1093/braincomms/fcaa113. PMID: 33215081; PMCID: PMC7660033.

[41] Francx W, Llera A, Mennes M, Zwiers MP, Faraone SV, Oosterlaan J, Heslenfeld D, Hoekstra PJ, Hartman CA, Franke B, Buitelaar JK, Beckmann CF. Integrated analysis of gray and white matter alterations in attention-deficit/hyperactivity disorder. Neuroimage Clin. 2016 Mar 4;11:357-367. doi: 10.1016/j.nicl.2016.03.005. PMID: 27298764; PMCID: PMC4893015.

[42] McLeod KR, Langevin LM, Dewey D, Goodyear BG. Atypical within- and between-hemisphere motor network functional connections in children with developmental coordination disorder and attention-deficit/hyperactivity disorder. Neuroimage Clin. 2016 Jun 28;12:157-64. doi: 10.1016/j.nicl.2016.06.019. PMID: 27419066; PMCID: PMC4936600.

[43] Hong J, Park BY, Cho HH, Park H. Age-related connectivity differences between attention deficit and hyperactivity disorder patients and typically developing subjects: a resting-state functional MRI study. Neural Regen Res. 2017 Oct;12(10):1640-1647. doi: 10.4103/1673-5374.217339. PMID: 29171429; PMCID: PMC5696845.

[44] Fan LY, Gau SS, Chou TL. Neural correlates of inhibitory control and visual processing in youths with attention deficit hyperactivity disorder: a counting Stroop functional MRI study. Psychol Med. 2014 Sep;44(12):2661-71. doi: 10.1017/S0033291714000038. Epub 2014 Jan 22. PMID: 24451066.

[45] Nugiel T, Roe MA, Engelhardt LE, Mitchell ME, Zheng A, Church JA. Pediatric ADHD symptom burden relates to distinct neural activity across executive function domains. Neuroimage Clin. 2020;28:102394. doi: 10.1016/j.nicl.2020.102394. Epub 2020 Aug 25. PMID: 32971467; PMCID: PMC7511724.

[46] Si FF, Liu L, Li HM, Sun L, Cao QJ, Lu H, Wang YF, Qian QJ. Cortical Morphometric Abnormality and Its Association with Working

Memory in Children with Attention-Deficit/Hyperactivity Disorder. Psychiatry Investig. 2021 Jul;18(7):679-687. doi: 10.30773/pi.2020.0333. Epub 2021 Jul 22. PMID: 34340276; PMCID: PMC8328834.

[47] Wu ZM, Llera A, Hoogman M, Cao QJ, Zwiers MP, Bralten J, An L, Sun L, Yang L, Yang BR, Zang YF, Franke B, Beckmann CF, Mennes M, Wang YF. Linked anatomical and functional brain alterations in children with attention-deficit/hyperactivity disorder. Neuroimage Clin. 2019;23:101851. doi: 10.1016/j.nicl.2019.101851. Epub 2019 May 4. PMID: 31077980; PMCID: PMC6514365.

[48] Duan K, Jiang W, Rootes-Murdy K, Schoenmacker GH, Arias-Vasquez A, Buitelaar JK, Hoogman M, Oosterlaan J, Hoekstra PJ, Heslenfeld DJ, Hartman CA, Calhoun VD, Turner JA, Liu J. Gray matter networks associated with attention and working memory deficit in ADHD across adolescence and adulthood. Transl Psychiatry. 2021 Mar 25;11(1):184. doi: 10.1038/s41398-021-01301-1. PMID: 33767139; PMCID: PMC7994833.

[49] Griffiths KR, Grieve SM, Kohn MR, Clarke S, Williams LM, Korgaonkar MS. Altered gray matter organization in children and adolescents with ADHD: a structural covariance connectome study. Transl Psychiatry. 2016 Nov 8;6(11):e947. doi: 10.1038/tp.2016.219. PMID: 27824356; PMCID: PMC5314130.

[50] Somandepalli K, Kelly C, Reiss PT, Zuo XN, Craddock RC, Yan CG, Petkova E, Castellanos FX, Milham MP, Di Martino A. Short-term test-retest reliability of resting state fMRI metrics in children with and without attention-deficit/hyperactivity disorder. Dev Cogn Neurosci. 2015 Oct;15:83-93. doi: 10.1016/j.dcn.2015.08.003. Epub 2015 Aug 11. PMID: 26365788; PMCID: PMC6989828.

[51] Cupertino RB, Soheili-Nezhad S, Grevet EH, Bandeira CE, Picon FA, Tavares MEA, Naaijen J, van Rooij D, Akkermans S, Vitola ES, Zwiers MP, Rovaris DL, Hoekstra PJ, Breda V, Oosterlaan J, Hartman CA, Beckmann CF, Buitelaar JK, Franke B, Bau CHD, Sprooten E. Reduced fronto-striatal volume in attention-deficit/hyperactivity disorder in two cohorts across the lifespan. Neuroimage Clin. 2020;28:102403. doi: 10.1016/j.nicl.2020.102403. Epub 2020 Aug 28. PMID: 32949876; PMCID: PMC7502360.

[52] Qian X, Loo BRY, Castellanos FX, Liu S, Koh HL, Poh XWW, Krishnan R, Fung D, Chee MW, Guan C, Lee TS, Lim CG, Zhou J. Brain-

computer-interface-based intervention re-normalizes brain functional network topology in children with attention deficit/hyperactivity disorder. Transl Psychiatry. 2018 Aug 10;8(1):149. doi: 10.1038/s41398-018-0213-8. PMID: 30097579; PMCID: PMC6086861.

[53] Bleich-Cohen M, Gurevitch G, Carmi N, Medvedovsky M, Bregman N, Nevler N, Elman K, Ginou A, Zangen A, Ash EL. A functional magnetic resonance imaging investigation of prefrontal cortex deep transcranial magnetic stimulation efficacy in adults with attention deficit/hyperactive disorder: A double blind, randomized clinical trial. Neuroimage Clin. 2021;30:102670. doi: 10.1016/j.nicl.2021.102670. Epub 2021 Apr 18. PMID: 34215144; PMCID: PMC8102620.

[54] Frodl T, Skokauskas N. Meta-analysis of structural MRI studies in children and adults with attention deficit hyperactivity disorder indicates treatment effects. Acta Psychiatr Scand. 2012 Feb;125(2):114-26. doi: 10.1111/j.1600-0447.2011.01786.x. Epub 2011 Nov 28. PMID: 22118249.

[55] Zhou R, Wang J, Han X, Ma B, Yuan H, Song Y. Baicalin regulates the dopamine system to control the core symptoms of ADHD. Mol Brain. 2019 Feb 8;12(1):11. doi: 10.1186/s13041-019-0428-5. PMID: 30736828; PMCID: PMC6368814.

[56] Iravani B, Arshamian A, Fransson P, Kaboodvand N. Whole-brain modelling of resting state fMRI differentiates ADHD subtypes and facilitates stratified neuro-stimulation therapy. Neuroimage. 2021 May 1;231:117844. doi: 10.1016/j.neuroimage.2021.117844. Epub 2021 Feb 10. PMID: 33577937.

[57] Kilpatrick LA, Joshi SH, O'Neill J, Kalender G, Dillon A, Best KM, Narr KL, Alger JR, Levitt JG, O'Connor MJ. Cortical gyrification in children with attention deficit-hyperactivity disorder and prenatal alcohol exposure. Drug Alcohol Depend. 2021 Aug 1;225:108817. doi: 10.1016/j.drugalcdep.2021.108817. Epub 2021 Jun 18. PMID: 34171826; PMCID: PMC8445068.

[58] Yadav SK, Bhat AA, Hashem S, Nisar S, Kamal M, Syed N, Temanni MR, Gupta RK, Kamran S, Azeem MW, Srivastava AK, Bagga P, Chawla S, Reddy R, Frenneaux MP, Fakhro K, Haris M. Genetic variations influence brain changes in patients with attention-deficit hyperactivity disorder. Transl Psychiatry. 2021 Jun 5;11(1):349. doi: 10.1038/s41398-021-01473-w. PMID: 34091591; PMCID: PMC8179928.

[59] Klein M, Onnink M, van Donkelaar M, Wolfers T, Harich B, Shi Y, Dammers J, Arias-Vásquez A, Hoogman M, Franke B. Brain imaging genetics in ADHD and beyond - Mapping pathways from gene to disorder at different levels of complexity. Neurosci Biobehav Rev. 2017 Sep;80:115-155. doi: 10.1016/j.neubiorev.2017.01.013. Epub 2017 Jan 31. PMID: 28159610; PMCID: PMC6947924.

[60] Zhou P, Wolraich ML, Cao AH, Jia FY, Liu B, Zhu L, Liu Y, Li X, Li C, Peng B, Yang T, Chen J, Cheng Q, Li T, Chen L. Adjuvant effects of vitamin A and vitamin D supplementation on treatment of children with attention-deficit/hyperactivity disorder: a study protocol for a randomised, double-blinded, placebo-controlled, multicentric trial in China. BMJ Open. 2021 Jun 16;11(6):e050541. doi: 10.1136/bmjopen-2021-050541. PMID: 34135055; PMCID: PMC8211063.

[61] Zhou Z, Zhou ZY, Kellar SS, Sikirica V, Xie J, Grebla R. Treatment patterns among adults with ADHD receiving long-acting therapy. Am J Manag Care. 2018 Jul;24(8 Spec No.):SP329-SP337. PMID: 30020748.

[62] Vander Stoep A, McCarty CA, Zhou C, Rockhill CM, Schoenfelder EN, Myers K. The Children's Attention-Deficit Hyperactivity Disorder Telemental Health Treatment Study: Caregiver Outcomes. J Abnorm Child Psychol. 2017 Jan;45(1):27-43. doi: 10.1007/s10802-016-0155-7. PMID: 27117555; PMCID: PMC5083233.

[63] Cohen R, Senecky Y, Shuper A, Inbar D, Chodick G, Shalev V, Raz R. Prevalence of epilepsy and attention-deficit hyperactivity (ADHD) disorder: a population-based study. J *Child Neurol.* 2013 Jan;28(1):120-3. doi: 10.1177/0883073812440327. Epub 2012 May 1. PMID:22550087.

Chapter 6
Neuroimaging Application in Drug Dependence

Abstract

The purposes of this chapter were to identify brain neural correlates of clinical data including drug dependence, with advanced multiparametric imaging quantification including fALFF/ReHo/VMHC, ICA-DR and dFNC methods. Significant negative associations between functional imaging metrics (including fALFF/ReHo/VMHC as well as intra-/inter- network functional connectivities identified with ICA-DR algorithms) and phenotypic data (such as dependence and time of use) were identified in multiple brain regions, including the ventral striatum, insular, cerebellum, temporal cortex and orbitofrontal cortex together with hypothalamus and ventromedial prefrontal cortex. Education and handcraft experience showed some neuroprotection effects in several regions including the orbitofrontal, ventral striatum, hypothalamus, superior frontal and temporal amygdala/hippocampus areas. Graph-theory based centrality showed significant correlations between binarized/weighted centrality degree and number of cigarettes per day as well as between weighted local degree centrality and number of cigarettes. Based on dFNC analysis, abnormally hyper-connectivities of connectograms in several states were identified including abnormally higher between-network dynamic correlations (close to 1) of state S4 for all the intra- and inter-network connections. The number of occurrence was relatively evenly distributed with close to mean value of 16% for all states (similar to the chess control group as in Chapter 1), while the distribution patterns of frequency and dwell time were similar to those of ADHD-AC type as illustrated in Chapter 5. Therapeutic strategies that target strengthening typical brain circuits in addiction such as CEN, DMN, SN and FPN/MN as well as thalamo-cortical connections might be effective for better brain inter-network modulation and dynamic facilitations with more regular behavior and better emotion/cognitive control.

Keywords: education, handedness score, neuroprotection, amygdala, thalamocortical network, centrality, number of cigarettes per day, drug dependence, time of use, therapeutic evaluation, multimodal imaging, multiparametric quantification, ventral striatum, insular, cerebellum, temporal cortex, orbitofrontal cortex, hypothalamus, ventromedial prefrontal cortex, graph theory, degree, centrality, hyper-connectivities, connectogram, state, therapeutic strategy, addiction, typical brain networks

1. Introduction

1.1. Overview

Numerous studies have been performed to investigate brain changes associated with drug addiction for better therapeutic and recovery effects. As an example, higher neural activity measured with fALFF in the striatum correlated with the age and duration of abstinent methamphetamine (MA) use that also had lower fALFF in the inferior frontal gyrus (IFG). ReHo values were lower in the striatum and additional regions of anterior cingulate cortex (ACC), sensorimotor area and precuneus in MA users compared to controls [1]. These regions with lower ReHo and fALFF including ACC, striatal caudate together with orbitofrontal cortex (OFC), ventrolateral prefrontal cortex (vlPFC) and ventromedial prefrontal cortex (vmPFC) also showed neural reactivity following the reward-related cues in cocaine withdrawal participants [2]. Moreover, the activation in the IFG correlated negatively with lifetime alcohol use episodes during the breathing load and activation in the parahippocampus gyrus (PHG) correlated with cannabis and alcohol use, possibly for negative reinforcements in the adolescents with substance use [3]. The cannabis use disorders (CUD) showed disrupted hyper-activations in several regions involving craving and reward; for instance, increased activations in the ventral striatum, pallidum and putamen, anterior insular cortex, supplementary motor area (SMA), angular gyrus and superior frontal gyrus (SFG) were indicated with the cannabis odor cues. While in the CUD group, these activations in specific regions of insula, ACC and occipital cortex related to the self-reported craving scores [4]. Based on connectome, dynamic functional connectivity between central executive network (CEN) and ventral striatum was increased during the cannabis cue exposure task, and was also strongly associated with subjective craving score [5]. The dysregulation in frontostriatal circuit for cognitive process and reward response with dissociable contributions in subjects during even short duration of use might explain the substance-specific behaviors and high sensitivities of these neural alterations in substance users such as CUD [6]. Some of the frontal networks were also involved in the general cost and risky decision making procedure including the insula and vmPFC circuits, while the subcortical striatum co-activated with the temporal amygdala and hippocampus regions as part of the memory/emotion/planning evaluation progress [7, 8].

Exposure to cannabis-cues may trigger cravings in regular CUD and elicit greater than normal functional activations in several key regions, including the aforementioned striatum and frontal cortex such as ACC, and additional parietal cortex, temporal hippocampus/amygdala, thalamus and occipital region [9]. Especially for the long-term CUD, hyper-responsivity and specificity in the ACC/striatum/OFC and ventral tegmental area (VTA) were demonstrated for natural reward cue in comparison to controls, indicating disrupted natural-reward processes and sensitization loss of mesocorticolimbic circuit following drug use [10, 11]. The motor–related regions including the precentral gyrus

(PCG) and SMA as well as insula (relating to sensorimotor function, olfactory stimuli, attention and salience processing in addition to social emotion) showed abnormally higher activation in the strong incentive win vs. neutral conditions, and correlated positively with cocaine craving questionnaire (CCQ) score [12, 13]. Also the cannabis cue-related activity in the insula and ACC was associated with CCQ while medial OFC activity was related to the years of use, together with the usual high activities in the ventral striatum and insula/amygdala [14]. Dynamic functional connectivity based classification identified connectivities of visual network (VN), CEN/DMN, sensorimotor cortex, insula and amygdala as the most significant imaging features with 95% accuracy [15]. Compared to non-dependent cannabis users, dependent users showed functional connectivity changes in the reward network seeded from the ventral striatum that followed neural response in the hippocampus and ACC during repeated cannabis exposure [16]. Investigation of heroin maintenance treatment identified lower connectivity between amygdala and fusiform as well as between amygdala and OFC, and the inter-regional amygdala functional alterations correlated with stress response and levels of craving [17]. Furthermore, during inhibitory control task, smoking abstinence showed less right insula and putamen activation [18]. Also weaker connectivity between posterior insula and primary sensorimotor was associated with relapse vulnerability, while insula functional connectivity linked to smoking cessation likelihood [19].

In the substance-dependent brain, large-scale network communication efficiency was lower via small-worldness analysis, indicating loss of inter-regional topology and also loss of inhibition as one of the drug seeking behaviors [20]. Also during acute nicotine abstinence, using the time varying functional connectivity (TVFC) analysis, both between-network modulation (temporal flexibility) and within-network variability (spatiotemporal diversity) were decreased, and these deficits related to clinical behavior symptoms [21]. In addition, based on graph theoretical metrics, the temporal flexibility was diminished together with compensated increased spatiotemporal diversity in majorities of neural networks in CUD such as CEN and DMN [22]. At the inter-network connectivity level, decreased functional connectivity between SN and FPN in smokers compared to nonsmokers was reported with additional corticocerebellar and subcortical-cerebellar smoke state-dependent network differences [23]. Moreover, inverse coupling between DMN and CEN was increased after nicotine replacement pharma-cotherapy, and these inter- and intra- network changes including additional CEN and reward systems were associated with the withdrawal symptom improvement [24]. Also negative coupling between FPN and prefrontal-limbic circuitry was associated with better self-control and delayed substance use onset in adolescents based on fMRI independent component analysis (ICA) method [25]. Typical network reconfiguration was reported such as among DMN, FPN, SN and VN that were transient and related to the addiction vulnerability and risky decision trait including reward dysfunction in alcoholism studies [26].

1.2. Objectives

Several types of drug dependence and their neural manifestation had been reviewed including abnormal brain circuits related to the reward, decision making and emotional control. The purposes of this chapter were to identify possible systematic brain neural correspondences for clinical data of drug dependence, with advanced multiparametric imaging quantification including fALFF/ReHo/VMHC, ICA-DR and dFNC.

2. Methods

2.1. Participants

Imaging data of 29 cocaine dependence individuals were provided by the New York University and downloaded with approval from the NITRC database (http://fcon_1000.projects.nitrc.org/indi/retro/nyuCocaine.html). All cocaine-dependent participants met the DSM-IV criteria (also within 1 year period of imaging study participation), with abstaining for longer than 2 weeks and screened at the time of MRI scan [27]. Demographic information of participants included: age of 37.2±9.5 years, 3 females (10%), education level of 4.0±0.9 (college level), handedness score of 81.3±27.4, number of cigarettes per day was 14.6±9.4 with 17 smokers, estimated years since first use of 13.3±9.5 and years of drug dependence was 6.8±6.5.

2.2. Iaging Parameters and Data Processing

MRI experiments were performed using the 3T scanner with standardized imaging protocols. The 3D MPRAGE sequence was run with TR/TI/TE=2530/1100/3.25 ms, flip angle=7°, matrix size=256 x 256 x 128, resolution=1 x 1.3 x 1.3 mm^3. For the resting-state (RS)-fMRI data acquired under relaxing condition, a conventional gradient-echo EPI sequence (TR/TE=2000/15 msec, flip angle=90°, number of volumes=180, spatial resolution=3 x 3 x 4 mm^3) was utilized.

The processed MRI and fMRI images including fALFF, ReHo, VMHC ICA-DR, and graph-theory based degree centrality metrics were downloaded. The 20 ICA-DR components (DR0-DR19) included typical functional neural networks such as DMN, SN, MN, VN, FPN, CEN and thalamocortical connection patterns. Relatively new dFNC algorithm was implemented to the preprocessed fMRI data for deriving the connectograms, dynamic dwell time and frequency/occupancy parameters. Quantitative correlations between functional as well as structural together with structural/ micro-structural imaging results and phenotypic scales were also performed to examine the associations of cognitive/behavior tests with neural activity/connectivity/network metrics [28-30].

3. Results

Significant functional imaging correlations with phenotypic data including fALFF, ReHo and VMHC fMRI metrics were present in Figure 1. Strong negative correlations ($P<0.05$) between frontal fALFF and cigarettes per day as well as between posterior parietal/cerebellar VMHC and cigarettes per day were found (Figure 1A). However, positive correlations between thalamo-cerebellar/insular ReHo and cigarettes per day existed on the other hand. Significant negative correlation between temporal fALFF and estimated years of dependence was revealed, together with the negative association between cerebellar/temporal/hippocampal/ lateral occipital VMHC and years of dependence (Figure 1B). On the other hand, positive associations with dependence also existed for the orbitofrontal including olfactory ReHo synchrony and frontoparietal/motor fALFF neural activity. Negative associations were observed between temporal/occipital/basal ganglia VMHC and estimated years since first use, as well as for the cerebellar VMHC/ ReHo/ fALFF values (Figure 1C).

Strong associations of functional images of fALFF/ReHo/VMHC and age in years, education level and handedness score were displayed in Figure 2 A-C respectively. Negative correlations between age and VMHC in the cerebellum, temporal cortex including hippocampus/ parahippocampal gyrus/amygdala/ middle temporal gyrus/ superior temporal regions, inferior parietal area, visual cortex including calcarine, lingual, precuneus and cuneus, subcortical putamen and pallidum, anterior thalamus were observed in Figure 2A. In addition, negative correlations between age and ReHo in the cerebellum but positive correlations between fALFF in the orbitofrontal cortex including olfactory tract and frontal pole as well as left motor area and age also existed. On the other hand, negative correlations between fALFF in the cerebellum, inferior/superior temporal/calcarine regions and subject age were also presented. Positive correlations between education levels and fALFF neural activity in several regions including the orbitofrontal cortex, cerebellum, thalamus, amygdala, putamen, insula and basal ganglia are shown in Figure 2B, while negative associations between education level and fALFF in the distributed regions of motor, parietal and superior frontal region were found as well. Negative correlations between education level and ReHo in the insular, inferior frontal and motor areas existed additionally. Figure 2C showed the positive associations between handedness score and ReHo values in the orbitofrontal, medial prefrontal and superior frontal regions. In contrast, negative associations between handedness score and ReHo values in the superior temporal, small motor and supplementary motor areas, posterior visual and cerebellum regions were exhibited. Further positive relationship between handedness score and fALFF in the orbitofrontal and superior frontal regions were observed. While negative correlations between handedness score and fALFF activity in small distributed clusters of insular, hippocampus/parahippocampus and calcarine were found as well. And negative associations were also found between handedness score and VMHC values in the visual, subcallosal cortex, anterior putamen and insula, rolandic operculum and orbitofrontal regions.

Negative associations between ICA-DR components (earlier components of 0-10) and cigarettes per day were presented in Figure

3a. For instance, negative associations were found between number of cigarettes per day and fMRI-based inter- and intra- network connectivities of the ventral striatum, hypothalamus, orbitofrontal cortex, anterior insula and visual circuits. Positive correlations existed for the small clusters in the cerebellum, thalamus and medial/superior frontal area as illustrated in Figure 3a. For the later ICA-DR components, negative associations were further found between number of cigarettes per day and network connectivity of the anterior temporal, striatum and medial orbitofrontal region as well as the supplementary motor/parietal areas and superior frontal clusters (Figure 3b). Positive correlations also existed for the small clusters in the cerebellum, posterior temporal segment and visual cortex.

Figure 4a showed negative associations between ICA-DR components (earlier components of 0-11) and estimated years since first use. For instance, negative associations between years since first use and network connectivity of the cerebellum, left orbitofrontal cortex, medial and middle temporal, occipital and insular regions were identified. Positive correlations existed for the small clusters in the hypothalamus/ subcallosal cortex and superior temporal/frontal areas. And Figure 4b illustrated the negative associations between ICA-DR later components of 12-19 and years since first use; especially for the network connectivity of cerebellum, right insular and parietal region. Positive correlations existed for the orbitofrontal, right media frontal, superior frontal and inferior parietal regions as well.

Then Figure 5a showed negative associations between ICA-DR components (earlier components of 0-10) and estimated years of dependence. For instance, negative associations were present between years of dependence and network connectivity of the medial orbitofrontal cortex, frontal pole, olfactory cortex, striatum including ventral striatum and left caudate, cerebellum and small basal ganglia areas together with the primary visual regions. Figure 5b displayed negative associations between ICA-DR components (later components of 11-18) and years of dependence. For instance, negative associations between years of dependence and network connectivity of cerebellum, right insula, ventromedial orbitofrontal cortex including the subcallosal cortex and temporal/lateral occipital regions were identified. And network connectivities of the ventral striatum, middle frontal cluster, hypothalamus and inferior parietal regions correlated positively with years of dependence.

Significant correlations between number of cigarettes per day and metrics of centrality based on graph theory analysis were discovered, including the binarized weighted centrality degree (R=0.67 and P=0.02) and weighted local functional connectivity degree (R=0.60, P=0.04) (Figure 6). Compared to conventional normal connectogram, hyper-connectivities in several states including S4, S3 and S6 were exhibited in Figure 7. Finally, the correlation map also showed abnormally higher correlations; for instance, close to 1 pattern for all inter-network correlation coefficiencies of state S4 were identified. Number of occurrence with bootstrap statistics showed relatively evenly distributed values for all states (15-22% for each state, lower in states 4-6 and highest in S3 in Figure 8A), similar to the control group in Chapter 1 Figure 4. Mean frequency and dwell time of six states were displayed in Figure 8B, with relatively higher dwell time in S1, S4 and S5 and lower in S3 and S6. The distribution pattern of dwell time was similar to that of ADHD-AC type as illustrated in Chapter 5 Figure 7.

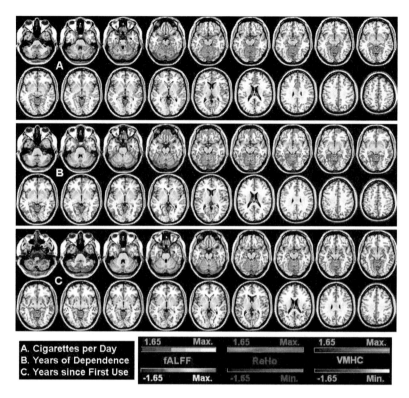

Figure 1. *Significant functional imaging correlations with phenotypic data including fALFF, ReHo and VMHC fMRI metrics. A: Strong negative correlations (P<0.05) between frontal fALFF and cigarettes per day (green x-rain color) as well as between VMHC posterior parietal/cerebellar and cigarettes per day (red/yellow x-hot color) were identified. However, positive correlations between thalamo-cerebellar/insular ReHo and cigarettes per day existed (purple NIH-ice color). B: Significant negative correlations between temporal fALFF and estimated years of dependence were revealed as well as between cerebella/temporal/hippocampal /lateral occipital VMHC and years of dependence, but positive associations also existed between years of dependence and orbitofrontal including olfactory ReHo as well as frontoparietal/motor fALFF. C: Negative associations between temporal/occipital/basal ganglia VMHC and estimated years since first use were observed, as well as with the cerebellar VMHC/ ReHo/ fALFF.*

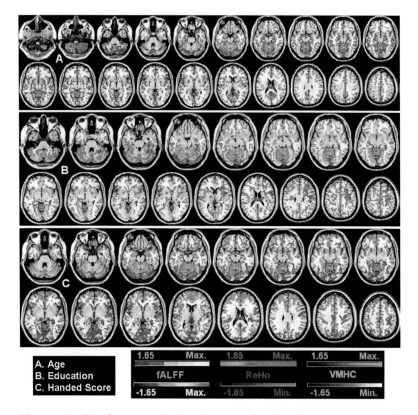

Figure 2. *Significant correlations between functional image z-scores of fALFF/ReHo/VMHC and age in years (A), education level (B) and handedness score (C). Negative associations of VMHC in the cerebellum, temporal regions including hippocampus/parahippocampal gyrus/amygdala/middle temporal gyrus/superior temporal region, inferior parietal area, visual cortex including calcarine, lingual, precuneus and cuneus, subcortical putamen and pallidum, anterior thalamus with age were observed as in A (x-hot color). Positive correlations between education levels and fALFF neural activity in several regions including the orbitofrontal cortex, cerebellum, thalamus, amygdala, putamen, insula and basal ganglia were found as in B (orange color). C. Positive associations were exhibited between handedness score and ReHo values in the orbitofrontal, medial prefrontal and superior frontal regions (purple color). In contrast, negative associations between handedness score and ReHo values in the superior temporal, small motor and supplementary motor areas, posterior visual and cerebellum*

regions existed (violet color). Further positive relationship between handedness score and fALFF values in the orbitofrontal and superior frontal regions were also observed (orange color).

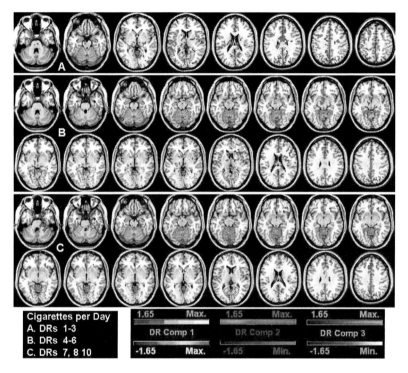

Figure 3a. *Negative associations between ICA-DR components (earlier components of 0-10) and cigarettes per day. For instance, negative associations were found between number of cigarettes per day and fMRI-based inter- and intra-network connectivities of the ventral striatum, hypothalamus, orbitofrontal cortex, anterior insula and visual circuits (x-rain and x-hot colors). Positive correlations existed for the small clusters in the cerebellum, thalamus and medial/superior frontal area (orange and purple colors).*

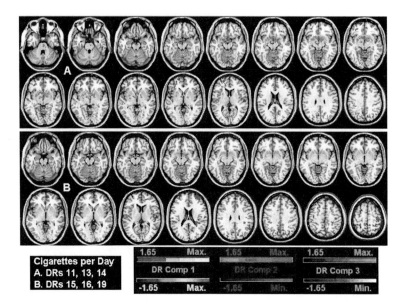

Figure 3b. *Negative associations between ICA-DR components (later components of 11-19) and cigarettes per day. For instance, negative associations were identified between number of cigarettes per day and network connectivity of the anterior temporal, striatum and medial orbitofrontal region as well as the supplementary motor/parietal areas and superior frontal clusters (x-rain, x-hot and violet colors). Positive correlations existed for the small clusters in the cerebellum, posterior temporal and visual cortex (orange color).*

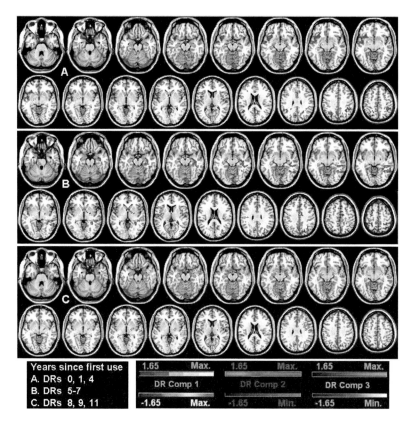

Figure 4a. *Negative associations between ICA-DR components (earlier components of 0-11) and estimated years since first use. For instance, negative associations between years since first use and network connectivities of the cerebellum, left orbitofrontal cortex, medial and middle temporal, occipital and insular regions were observed (x-rain and x-hot colors). Positive correlations existed for the small clusters in the hypothalamus/subcallosal cortex and superior temporal/frontal areas (orange and purple colors).*

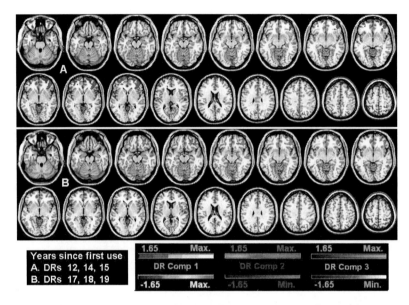

Figure 4b. *Negative associations between ICA-DR components (later components of 12-19) and years since first use. Negative associations between years since first use and network connectivity of cerebellum, right insular and parietal region were revealed (x-rain color). Positive correlations existed for the orbitofrontal, right media frontal, superior frontal and inferior parietal regions (orange and dark green colors in B).*

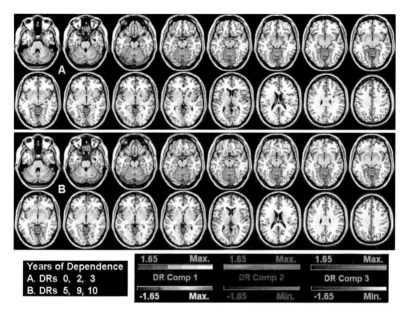

Figure 5a. *Negative associations between ICA-DR components (earlier components of 0-10) and estimated years of dependence. The negative associations between years of dependence and network connectivities of the medial orbitofrontal cortex, frontal pole, olfactory cortex, striatum including ventral striatum and left caudate, cerebellum and small basal ganglia areas together with the primary visual regions were found (x-rain, x-hot and violet colors).*

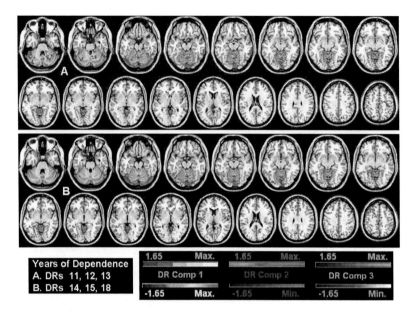

Figure 5b. *Negative associations between ICA-DR components (later components of 11-18) and years of dependence. Negative associations between years of dependence and network connectivity of cerebellum, right insula, ventromedial orbitofrontal including the subcallosal cortex and temporal/lateral occipital regions were identified (x-rain, x-hot and violet colors). Positive correlations existed for the ventral striatum, middle frontal cluster, hypothalamus and inferior parietal regions (orange and purple colors).*

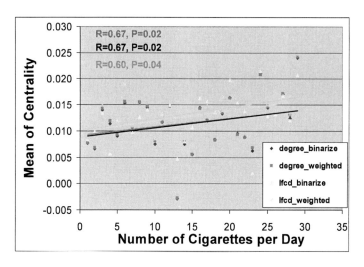

Figure 6. *Significant correlations between metrics of centrality and number of cigarettes per day (NCPD), including R=0.67 and P=0.02 between binarized/weighted centrality degree and NCPD as well as R=0.60, P=0.04 between weighted local functional connectivity degree (lfcd) centrality and NCPD.*

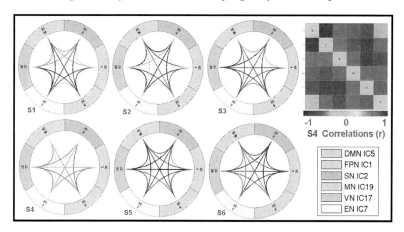

Figure 7. *Dynamic connectogram of six typical networks and inter-correlations from six states. Compared to conventional normal connectogram, hyper-connectivities in several states including S4, S3 and S6 were exhibited. As an example, the correlation map on the right top panel also showed abnormally higher correlations (close to 1) of state S4 for all the inter-network connections.*

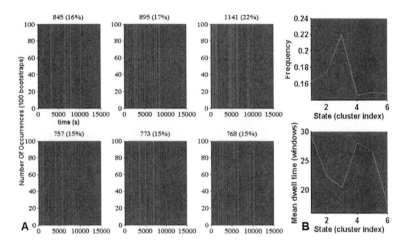

Figure 8. *A: Number of occurrence with bootstrap statistics showed relatively evenly distributed values for all states (15-22% for each state, lower in states 4-6 and highest in S3). Mean frequency (as in A), and mean dwell time of six states were displayed in panel B, with relatively higher dwell time in S1, S4 and S5 and lower in S3 and S6.*

4. Discussion

4.1. Summary of Results

Significant and expected negative associations between functional imaging such as fALFF/ReHo/VMHC and phenotypic data included: 1. *Cigarettes per day* correlated with frontal fALFF and posterior parietal/cerebellar VMHC; 2. *Years of dependence* correlated with temporal fALFF and cerebellar/temporal/hippocampal/lateral occipital VMHC; and 3. *Estimated years since first use* linked to temporal/occipital VMHC and cerebellar VMHC/ ReHo/ fALFF. And significant associations between functional imaging such as fALFF/ReHo/VMHC values with behavioral data (age/education level/handedness score) included: 1. *Age* correlated negatively with VMHC in the cerebellum, temporal regions including hippocampus/ parahippocampal gyrus/amygdala/middle temporal gyrus/superior temporal gyrus/inferior parietal area, visual cortex including calcarine, lingual, precuneus and cuneus, subcortical putamen and pallidum and anterior thalamus; indicating age-related memory and visuospaital abilities decline in drug users. 2. *Education level* correlated positively with fALFF neural activity in several regions including the orbitofrontal cortex, cerebellum, thalamus, amygdala, putamen, insula and basal ganglia; while these regions played important roles in reward perception, social values, motor function and internal emotion control. 3. *Handedness score* correlated positively with ReHo values in the all frontal regions including orbitofrontal/medial and superior segments as well as with fALFF in the orbitofrontal and superior frontal regions, indicating possible neural activity, synchrony and integration functionality improvement with more handcraft skills and practice.

Negative associations between intra-/inter- network functional connectivities identified with ICA-DR algorithms and phenotypic data included: 1. *between number of cigarettes per day* and network connectivities of ventral striatum, hypothalamus, orbitofrontal cortex, anterior insula and visual circuits as well as additional anterior temporal, striatum and medial orbitofrontal region, supplementary motor/parietal areas and superior frontal clusters; 2. *between estimated years since first use* and network connectivities of the cerebellum, left orbitofrontal cortex, medial and middle temporal, occipital and insular regions as well as additional parietal region; 3. *between years of dependence* and network connectivity of the medial orbitofrontal cortex, frontal pole, olfactory cortex, striatum including ventral striatum and left caudate, cerebellum and small basal ganglia areas together with primary visual regions as well as additional insula, ventromedial orbitofrontal cortex including the subcallosal cortex and temporal/lateral occipital regions. These typical regions including orbitofrontal cortex, ventral striatum, insular, temporal amygdala/hippocampus and hypothalamus with strong relationships to dosage of addiction and severity effects were in agreement with published neuroimaging findings of reward circuit and emotion-memory pathway.

Graph-theory based centrality showed significant correlations between number of cigarettes per day and binarized weighted local and centrality degrees. Based on dFNC analysis, abnormally hyper-connectivities of connectograms in several states were identified including abnormally higher correlations (close to 1) of state S4 for all the connections. The numbers of occurrence were relatively evenly distributed with close to mean value of 16% for all states (similar to the chess control group as in Chapter 1), while the distribution patterns of frequency and mean dwell time were similar to those of ADHD-AC type as illustrated in Chapter 5. The hyperconnectivity and dynamic state shifting disturbance indicated possible loss of reward sensitivity, drug craving and seeking behavior, addiction-trapped and risky decision-making problems in drug users.

4.2 Multimodal Imaging Findings

Neuroimaging studies including MRI and PET for drug cue reactivity modulation mapping and associated addiction severity prediction as well as treatment effects evaluation had been performed for better design of treatment and prevention [31]. For instance, gray matter volume (GMV) was reduced in several areas including lateral frontal, parietal, occipital cortices and cerebellum in the active cocaine users compared to controls, and linked to the impulsivity and delayed reward measures in frontal and posterior parietal cortices [32]. Structural volume asymmetry of the ventral striatum was associated with the dependence level that was disrupted in the substance users such as alcohol and nicotine [33]. The neural correlates of visually-cued cannabis craving were further investigated with results showing significant correlations between activations in the limbic (amygdala and hippocampus) and paralimbic (superior temporal pole) systems as well as between visual cortex activity and craving score [34]. The genetic rs10799590 allele was a robustly protective CNIH3 SNP in opioid dependence, and displayed significant amygdala habituation to threat-related facial expression [35]. In addition, higher activation of hypothalamus was reported in response to both cocaine and food cues, and correlated with the CCQ and days of cocaine use in prior month [36]. Finally, cortical thickness increased in the marijuana users compared to controls in the entorhinal cortex, and was related to the starting years of use. While cortical thickness in the frontal and temporal regions linked negatively to lifetime marijuana use [37].

4.3. Review of Therapeutic Effects and Related Findings

Brain function improvement that could adjust and improve goal-directed control behavior in regions including frontal cortex to reduce drug craving and use dependence as well as normalization of striatal reward function with deep brain stimulation are some targeted therapeutic interventions for opioid and metham-phetamine use disorders [38]. Reduced learning rate that led to poor instrument learning performance was revealed in CUD patients, as indicated with disrupted striatal and temporal functional activation and structural connectivity deterioration in the goal-directed control network [39]. Perfusion-based cerebral blood flow metric identified several addiction-related regions including the DMN, CEN, contextual memory and behavioral control, with acceptable accuracy for distinguishing cocaine-dependent participants from controls [40]. Brain hypoactivity was exhibited in cocaine addiction with the compulsive use behavior but not the amount consumed, and might be used for distinguishing nonaddict-like from addict-like CUD subgroups in rats model [41]. Also lipidomic phospholipid abundance level was lower in the hippocampus region of rat brain, indicating possible cocaine-induced lipid remodeling and homeostasis regulation [42]. And emotional network connectivity seeding from the amygdala was increased in the prenatal cocaine exposure aged group, but decreased in the control group compared to younger age [43]. Additionally, during cannabis approach avoidance training (CAAT) as a cognitive bias modification intervention, decreased activities in the amygdala and medial prefrontal cortex were identified compared to CAAT-sham [44]. Furthermore, some traditional Chinese medicine such as approved Fukang tablet as well as herbs including Rhizoma corydalis (Yanhusuo) and Radix Ginseng had been effective for reinforcing energy and removing toxicity [45]. Another traditional Chinese herb, Uncaria rhynchophylla (Goteng) together with Gastrodin were neuroprotective and inhibitory of drug dependence, and could help maintaining internal homeostasis integrity and further improved neuroregeneration and neuroplasticity [46].

4.4 Conclusion

In conclusion, significant associations between phenotypic data such as dependence/dosage and quantitative imaging metrics including neural activity and connectivity in typical orbitofrontal, ventral striatum, insula, hypothalamus, temporal cortex and cerebellum were revealed in this chapter. Abnormally higher centrality and hyper-connectivities of dynamic network regulation were also observed, that might be related to the severity of addiction and loss of inhibition in substance users as reflected by strong association with number of cigarettes per day. Our previous chapters 1-4 had demonstrated the beneficial effects of arts and science in professionals and experts such as chess masters, music/ mathematical practice, early college learning experience, daily skills and culture-based exercise on brain function facilitation, including neuroplasticity gain and enhancements of memory and attention, reward perception, emotion regulation and social values as well as intelligent decision making and efficient coordination systems.

Summary of imaging differences and phenotypic correlational results of all six chapters are listed in Table 1 and Table 2 respectively. As always emphasized, higher education level and better handcraft skills might help improve brain neural activity and temporal synchrony/integration in the mesocorticolimbic regions including orbitofrontal cortex, ventral striatum, amygdala/ hippocampus, superior frontal and visual cortex, and thus reduce relapse vulnerability as well as correct systematic reward and decision disruption in drug users. Therapeutic strategies that target strengthening brain circuits of addicted individuals such as CEN, DMN, SN and FPN/MN together with thalamo-cortical connections might be effective for better brain inter-network modulation and dynamic functionality optimization with more regular behavior and enhanced emotion/cognitive control.

Comp. Results	VBM (GMD)	VMHC	ICA-DR	SMW	ReHo/fALFF	dFNC
Chess	Higher in SFG, caudate, cerebellum, occipito-parietal junction, dorsal medial thalamus, SMA and OFC	Higher in temporal, SFG, MPFC, visual, hypothalamus, basal ganglia and cerebellar regions	Higher in VN, thalamocortical, DMN-MPFC, SN-superior temporal, and SFG	Higher absolute local but lower relative global efficiencies, slightly lower SMW factor	Higher global mean Z-values of ReHo, fALFF and sub-bands S4/S5, VMHC	Higher SN-CEN, SN-DMN, FPN-MN and VN-DMN; longer mean dwell time
Music	Higher VMHC in MPFC, DLPFC, ACC, SMA, striatum, superior temporal, occipital and cerebellum regions		Higher FPN, DMN, fronto-VN, thalamo-temporal, inter-SN & DMN; higher local/lower global SMW			Higher temporal dynamics at task conditions.
Counting	Higher VMHC in frontoparietal regions (FPN) including IPS and MPFC as well as temporal and SFG		Higher SN-DMN, DMN-CEN, FPN, VN-MN, temporal-DMN and frontal-DMN; higher local/lower global SMW		Lower VMHC and fALFF and sub-bands S5 in three task conditions compared to resting state	Higher mean dwell times under counting and resting state vs. the music and memory tasks
Memory	Higher VMHC in memory structure such as hippocampus, frontal pole, PCC, DLPFC and parietal regions		Higher DMN-FPN, SN-MN, temporal-FPN, thalamo-temporal, higher small-worldness factor			

Comp. Results	VBM (GMD)	VMHC	ICA-DR	SMW	ReHo/fALFF	dFNC
ADHD-C	Abnormally higher in medial OFC, ACC, DMN (PCC & MPFC), cuneus, superior temporal region and SMA	Abnormally Higher in ACC, OFC, SMA, occipital cortex, cerebellum, thalamus, striatum, amygdala, temporal and basal ganglia	Lower in visuo-temporal, DMN, thalamic-occipital, FPN-VN and fronto-temporal networks; Higher visual, thalamo-temporal, CEN-DMN, FPN-CEN and VN-MN	Lowest relative local efficiency and small-worldness configuration factor, but highest absolute local efficiency	Slightly lower frontal neural activity but higher in the cerebellum; Higher synchrony in visuomotor areas but lower	Reversal dFNC pattern in AC and similar to epilepsy comorbid pattern; AC group tended to stay in lower dwell time states more often; dwell time was lower in AI & AC patients compared to TD
ADHD-I	Higher in caudate temporal, and cerebellum Lower in temporal, insular and motor	Higher in rectus, amygdala, ACC, hippocampus; Lower in superior temporal & lingual	Higher in small inferior parietal, caudate and MPFC; Lower in PCC and somatosensory cortex	Highest relative local efficiency, but lowest absolute local efficiency	putamen and cerebellum in AC vs. typically developed (TD) controls	

Summary Table 1. *Group comparison (Comp.) statistical difference results in Chapter 1 (Chess), chapter 2 (music/counting/memory tasks) and chapter 5 (ADHD). GMD=gray matter density; SFG=superior frontal gyrus; OFC=orbitofrontal cortex; SMA=supplementary motor area; ACC=anterior cingulate; MPFC=medial frontal cortex; DLPFC=dorsolateral prefrontal cortex; IPS=intra-parietal sulcus; PCC=posterior cingulate*

Corr. Results	Education-EI	Education-TS	Raven's CRT	Age	Movie	Addiction
fALFF	insula, hypothalamus, cuneus and MA	frontal, MA/SMA, thalamus, basal ganglia and temporoparietal regions	occipital, inferior and medial temporal, DLPFC, small caudate and thalamus	Negative aging effects of ReHo in superior temporal/ insula and fALFF in sensorimotor/ MA; positive for occipital VMHC/ fALFF/ReHo; higher VMHC in PCC, temporal and IPL longitudinally	Higher VMHC at inscape compared to rest and movie conditions; relatively higher movie/inscape fALFF neural activity compared to rest/flankers; similar dFNC and more session effects of ICA-DR network correlations; fALFF/VMHC linked to ISQ/ISQ2	OFC, ventral striatum (VST), insular, temporal amygdala/ hippocampus and hypothalamus neural activities/connectivit ies related to dosage of addiction, dependence and severity effects with abnormally high dFNC. Better education and handcraft skills linked positively to mesocorticolimbic regions including OFC/VST/hypothala mus/hippocampus for neural activity/ connectivity enhancement.
ReHo	Parietal and superior temporal clusters, premotor and MA	SFG and insular region; frontoparietal clusters and premotor/MA	OFC and SFG, insular, superior temporal and MA/SMA			
VMHC	ACC, OFC, occipital cortex and cerebellum	Cerebellum, medial temporal and parietal cortices	OFC, IFG, MPFC, PCC, SMA, superior temporal, occipital and cerebellum			

Corr. Results	Education-EI	Education-TS	Raven's CRT	Age	Movie	Addiction
VBM	OFC, cerebellum, insula, fusiform, cuneus, PCC, MPFC, caudate, putamen	temporal regions including hippocampus and parahippocampus, OFC, SFG, visual and sensorimotor areas	temporal, insula and cuneus regions	Age-related lower GMD in temporal, insula and cuneus	Regions in the medial OFC/SFG, middle temporal gyrus, IPS, MA, angular gyrus, premotor area and various subregions in visual cortex (V1-V5) showed larger between-session ICA-DR differences	OFC, ventral striatum (VST), insular, temporal amygdala/ hippocampus and hypothalamus neural activities/connectivities related to dosage of addiction, dependence and severity effects with abnormally high dFNC. Better education and handcraft skills linked positively to mesocorticolimbic regions including OFC/VST/hypothalamus/hippocampus for neural activity/ connectivity enhancement.
DTI	thalamic radiation, splenium of corpus callosum, internal capsule, cingulum, SLF/CST	cingulum, SLF, CST, uncinate fasciculus and major forceps	tracts of cingulum, hippocampus, thalamic radiation, internal capsule, uncinate fasciculus	AD/MD increased with age in internal capsule and CST		
SMW	increased global but decreased local efficiencies at time point (TP)3 compared to TP2 and TP1 with more efficient and optimal SMW topology after college educational training				increased local and global session efficiencies	

Summary Table 2. *Statistical imaging correlational (Corr.) results in Chapter 3 (EI and TS), chapter 4 (four conditions of movie, inscape, flankers and resting state) and chapter 6 (addiction). EI=emotional intelligence; TS=trait score; SFG=superior frontal gyrus; OFC=orbitofrontal cortex; MA=motor area; SMA=supplementary motor area; ACC=anterior cingulate; MPFC=medial frontal cortex; DLPFC=dorsolateral prefrontal cortex; IPS=intra-parietal sulcus; PCC=posterior cingulate; IPL=inferior parietal lobe; SLF=superior longitudinal fasciculus; CST=cortico-spinal tract*

References

[1] Xie A, Wu Q, Yang WFZ, Qi C, Liao Y, Wang X, Hao W, Tang YY, Liu J, Liu T, Tang J. Altered patterns of fractional amplitude of low-frequency fluctuation and regional homogeneity in abstinent methamphetamine-dependent users. Sci Rep. 2021 Apr 8;11(1):7705. doi: 10.1038/s41598-021-87185-z. PMID: 33833282; PMCID: PMC8032776.

[2] Denomme WJ, Shane MS. History of withdrawal modulates drug- and food-cue reactivity in cocaine dependent participants. Drug Alcohol Depend. 2020 Mar 1;208:107815. doi: 10.1016/j.drugalcdep. 2019.107815. Epub 2019 Dec 23. PMID: 31972520.

[3] May AC, Jacobus J, Stewart JL, Simmons AN, Paulus MP, Tapert SF. Do Adolescents Use Substances to Relieve Uncomfortable Sensations? A Preliminary Examination of Negative Reinforcement among Adolescent Cannabis and Alcohol Users. Brain Sci. 2020 Apr 5;10(4):214. doi: 10.3390/brainsci10040214. PMID: 32260480; PMCID: PMC7226193.

[4] Kleinhans NM, Sweigert J, Blake M, Douglass B, Doane B, Reitz F, Larimer M. FMRI activation to cannabis odor cues is altered in individuals at risk for a cannabis use disorder. Brain Behav. 2020 Oct;10(10):e01764. doi: 10.1002/brb3.1764. Epub 2020 Aug 30. PMID: 32862560; PMCID: PMC7559640.

[5] Yoo HB, Moya BE, Filbey FM. Dynamic functional connectivity between nucleus accumbens and the central executive network relates to chronic cannabis use. Hum Brain Mapp. 2020 Sep;41(13):3637-3654. doi: 10.1002/hbm.25036. Epub 2020 May 20. PMID: 32432821; PMCID: PMC7416060.

[6] Klugah-Brown B, Di X, Zweerings J, Mathiak K, Becker B, Biswal B. Common and separable neural alterations in substance use disorders: A coordinate-based meta-analyses of functional neuroimaging studies in humans. Hum Brain Mapp. 2020 Nov;41(16):4459-4477. doi: 10.1002/hbm.25085. Epub 2020 Sep 10. PMID: 32964613; PMCID: PMC7555084.

[7] Steward T, Juaneda-Seguí A, Mestre-Bach G, Martínez-Zalacaín I, Vilarrasa N, Jiménez-Murcia S, Fernández-Formoso JA, Veciana de Las Heras M, Custal N, Virgili N, Lopez-Urdiales R, García-Ruiz-de-

Gordejuela A, Menchón JM, Soriano-Mas C, Fernandez-Aranda F. What Difference Does it Make? Risk-Taking Behavior in Obesity after a Loss is Associated with Decreased Ventromedial Prefrontal Cortex Activity. J Clin Med. 2019 Sep 27;8(10):1551. doi: 10.3390/jcm8101551. PMID: 31569607; PMCID: PMC6832276.

[8] Goldman M, Szucs-Reed RP, Jagannathan K, Ehrman RN, Wang Z, Li Y, Suh JJ, Kampman K, O'Brien CP, Childress AR, Franklin TR. Reward-related brain response and craving correlates of marijuana cue exposure: a preliminary study in treatment-seeking marijuana-dependent subjects. J Addict Med. 2013 Jan-Feb;7(1):8-16. doi: 10.1097/ADM.0b013e318273863a.   PMID: 23188041;   PMCID: PMC3567235.)

[9] Sehl H, Terrett G, Greenwood LM, Kowalczyk M, Thomson H, Poudel G, Manning V, Lorenzetti V. Patterns of brain function associated with cannabis cue-reactivity in regular cannabis users: a systematic review of fMRI studies. Psychopharma-cology (Berl). 2021 Sep 10. doi: 10.1007/s00213-021-05973-x. Epub ahead of print. PMID: 34505940.

[10] Filbey FM, DeWitt SJ. Cannabis cue-elicited craving and the reward neurocircuitry. Prog Neuropsychopharmacol Biol Psychiatry. 2012 Jul 2;38(1):30-5. doi: 10.1016/j.pnpbp.2011.11.001. Epub 2011 Nov 9. PMID: 22100353; PMCID: PMC3623277.

[11] Filbey FM, Dunlop J, Ketcherside A, Baine J, Rhinehardt T, Kuhn B, DeWitt S, Alvi T. fMRI study of neural sensitization to hedonic stimuli in long-term, daily cannabis users. Hum Brain Mapp. 2016 Oct;37(10):3431-43. doi: 10.1002/hbm.23250. Epub 2016 May 11. PMID: 27168331; PMCID: PMC5012952.

[12] Zhornitsky S, Dhingra I, Le TM, Wang W, Li CR, Zhang S. Reward-Related Responses and Tonic Craving in Cocaine Addiction: An Imaging Study of the Monetary Incentive Delay Task. Int J Neuropsychopharmacol.   2021   Aug   20;24(8):634-644.   doi: 10.1093/ijnp/pyab016. PMID: 33822080; PMCID: PMC8378081.

[13] Uddin LQ, Nomi JS, Hébert-Seropian B, Ghaziri J, Boucher O. Structure and Function of the Human Insula. J Clin Neurophysiol. 2017 Jul;34(4):300-306. doi: 10.1097/WNP. 0000000000000377. PMID: 28644199; PMCID: PMC6032992.

[14] Wetherill RR, Childress AR, Jagannathan K, Bender J, Young KA, Suh JJ, O'Brien CP, Franklin TR. Neural responses to subliminally

presented cannabis and other emotionally evocative cues in cannabis-dependent individuals. Psychopharmacology (Berl). 2014 Apr;231(7):1397-407. doi: 10.1007/s00213-013-3342-z. Epub 2013 Nov 2. PMID: 24186078; PMCID: PMC6218642.

[15] Sakoglu U, Mete M, Esquivel J, Rubia K, Briggs R, Adinoff B. Classification of cocaine-dependent participants with dynamic functional connectivity from functional magnetic resonance imaging data. J Neurosci Res. 2019 Jul;97(7):790-803. doi: 10.1002/jnr.24421. Epub 2019 Apr 7. PMID: 30957276; PMCID: PMC6530930.

[16] Filbey FM, Dunlop J. Differential reward network functional connectivity in cannabis dependent and non-dependent users. Drug Alcohol Depend. 2014 Jul 1;140:101-11. doi: 10.1016/j.drugalcdep.2014.04.002. Epub 2014 Apr 13. PMID: 24838032; PMCID: PMC4349558.

[17] Schmidt A, Walter M, Gerber H, Seifritz E, Brenneisen R, Wiesbeck GA, Riecher-Rössler A, Lang UE, Borgwardt S. Normalizing effect of heroin maintenance treatment on stress-induced brain connectivity. Brain. 2015 Jan;138(Pt 1):217-28. doi: 10.1093/brain/awu326. Epub 2014 Nov 19. PMID: 25414039; PMCID: PMC4285192.

[18] Lesage E, Sutherland MT, Ross TJ, Salmeron BJ, Stein EA. Nicotine dependence (trait) and acute nicotinic stimulation (state) modulate attention but not inhibitory control: converging fMRI evidence from Go-Nogo and Flanker tasks. Neuropsychopharmacology. 2020 Apr;45(5):857-865. doi: 10.1038/s41386-020-0623-1. Epub 2020 Jan 29. PMID: 31995811; PMCID: PMC7075893.

[19] Addicott MA, Sweitzer MM, Froeliger B, Rose JE, McClernon FJ. Increased Functional Connectivity in an Insula-Based Network is Associated with Improved Smoking Cessation Outcomes. Neuropsychopharmacology. 2015 Oct;40(11):2648-56. doi: 10.1038/npp. 2015.114. Epub 2015 Apr 21. PMID: 25895453; PMCID: PMC4569957.

[20] Wang Z, Suh J, Li Z, Li Y, Franklin T, O'Brien C, Childress AR. A hyper-connected but less efficient small-world network in the substance-dependent brain. Drug Alcohol Depend. 2015 Jul 1;152:102-8. doi: 10.1016/j.drugalcdep.2015.04.015. Epub 2015 May 1. PMID: 25957794; PMCID: PMC4458212.

[21] Fedota JR, Ross TJ, Castillo J, McKenna MR, Matous AL, Salmeron BJ, Menon V, Stein EA. Time-Varying Functional Connectivity Decreases

as a Function of Acute Nicotine Abstinence. Biol Psychiatry Cogn Neurosci Neuroimaging. 2021 Apr;6(4):459-469. doi: 10.1016/j.bpsc. 2020.10.004. Epub 2020 Oct 19. PMID: 33436331; PMCID: PMC8035238.

[22] Zhang Y, Zhang S, Ide JS, Hu S, Zhornitsky S, Wang W, Dong G, Tang X, Li CR. Dynamic network dysfunction in cocaine dependence: Graph theoretical metrics and stop signal reaction time. Neuroimage Clin. 2018 Mar 16;18:793-801. doi: 10.1016/j.nicl.2018.03.016. PMID: 29876265; PMCID: PMC5988015.

[23] Yip SW, Lichenstein SD, Garrison K, Averill CL, Viswanath H, Salas R, Abdallah CG. Effects of Smoking Status and State on Intrinsic Connectivity. Biol Psychiatry Cogn Neurosci Neuroimaging. 2021 Feb 19:S2451-9022(21)00050-1. doi: 10.1016/j.bpsc.2021.02.004. Epub ahead of print. PMID: 33618016; PMCID: PMC8373998.

[24] Cole DM, Beckmann CF, Long CJ, Matthews PM, Durcan MJ, Beaver JD. Nicotine replacement in abstinent smokers improves cognitive withdrawal symptoms with modulation of resting brain network dynamics. Neuroimage. 2010 Aug 15;52(2):590-9. doi: 10.1016/ j.neuroimage.2010.04.251. Epub 2010 May 2. PMID: 20441798.

[25] Lee TH, Telzer EH. Negative functional coupling between the right fronto-parietal and limbic resting state networks predicts increased self-control and later substance use onset in adolescence. Dev Cogn Neurosci. 2016 Aug;20:35-42. doi: 10.1016/j.dcn.2016.06.002. Epub 2016 Jun 17. PMID: 27344035; PMCID: PMC4975996.

[26] Amico E, Dzemidzic M, Oberlin BG, Carron CR, Harezlak J, Goñi J, Kareken DA. The disengaging brain: Dynamic transitions from cognitive engagement and alcoholism risk. Neuroimage. 2020 Apr 1;209:116515. doi: 10.1016/j.neuroimage.2020.116515. Epub 2020 Jan 2. PMID:31904492.

[7] Kelly C, Zuo XN, Gotimer K, Cox CL, Lynch L, Brock D, Imperati D, Garavan H, Rotrosen J, Castellanos FX, Milham MP. Reduced interhemispheric resting state functional connectivity in cocaine addiction. Biol Psychiatry. 2011 Apr 1;69(7):684-92. doi: 10.1016/j.biopsych.2010.11.022. Epub 2011 Jan 20. PMID: 21251646; PMCID: PMC3056937.

[28] Zhou Y. *Joint Imaging Applications in General Neurodegenerative Disease: Parkinson's, Frontotemporal, Vascular Dementia and Autism.* Nova Science Publishers. 2021.

[29] Zhou Y. *Imaging and Multiomic Biomarker Applications: Advances in Early Alzheimer's Disease.* Nova Science Publishers. 2020.

[30] Zhou Y. *Typical Imaging in Atypical Parkinson's, Schizophrenia, Epilepsy and Asymptomatic Alzheimer's Disease.* Nova Science Publishers. 2021.

[31] Jasinska AJ, Stein EA, Kaiser J, Naumer MJ, Yalachkov Y. Factors modulating neural reactivity to drug cues in addiction: a survey of human neuroimaging studies. Neurosci Biobehav Rev. 2014 Jan;38:1-16. doi: 10.1016/j.neubiorev.2013.10.013. Epub 2013 Nov 6. PMID: 24211373; PMCID: PMC3913480.

[32] Meade CS, Bell RP, Towe SL, Hall SA. Cocaine-related alterations in fronto-parietal gray matter volume correlate with trait and behavioral impulsivity. Drug Alcohol Depend. 2020 Jan 1;206:107757. doi: 10.1016/j.drugalcdep.2019.107757. Epub 2019 Nov 20. PMID: 31805488; PMCID: PMC6980751.

[33] Cao Z, Ottino-Gonzalez J, Cupertino RB, Schwab N, Hoke C, Catherine O, Cousijn J, Dagher A, Foxe JJ, Goudriaan AE, Hester R, Hutchison K, Li CR, London ED, Lorenzetti V, Luijten M, Martin-Santos R, Momenan R, Paulus MP, Schmaal L, Sinha R, Sjoerds Z, Solowij N, Stein DJ, Stein EA, Uhlmann A, van Holst RJ, Veltman DJ, Wiers RW, Yücel M, Zhang S, Jahanshad N, Thompson PM, Conrod P, Mackey S, Garavan H. Mapping cortical and subcortical asymmetries in substance dependence: Findings from the ENIGMA Addiction Working Group. Addict Biol. 2021 Sep;26(5):e13010. doi: 10.1111/adb.13010. Epub 2021 Jan 28. PMID: 33508888; PMCID: PMC8317852.

[34] Charboneau EJ, Dietrich MS, Park S, Cao A, Watkins TJ, Blackford JU, Benningfield MM, Martin PR, Buchowski MS, Cowan RL. Cannabis cue-induced brain activation correlates with drug craving in limbic and visual salience regions: preliminary results. Psychiatry Res. 2013 Nov 30;214(2):122-31. doi: 10.1016/j.pscychresns.2013. 06.005. Epub 2013 Sep 12. PMID: 24035535; PMCID: PMC3904759.

[35] Nelson EC, Agrawal A, Heath AC, Bogdan R, Sherva R, Zhang B, Al-Hasani R, Bruchas MR, Chou YL, Demers CH, Carey CE, Conley ED, Fakira AK, Farrer LA, Goate A, Gordon S, Henders AK, Hesselbrock

V, Kapoor M, Lynskey MT, Madden PA, Moron JA, Rice JP, Saccone NL, Schwab SG, Shand FL, Todorov AA, Wallace L, Wang T, Wray NR, Zhou X, Degenhardt L, Martin NG, Hariri AR, Kranzler HR, Gelernter J, Bierut LJ, Clark DJ, Montgomery GW. Evidence of CNIH3 involvement in opioid dependence. Mol Psychiatry. 2016 May;21(5):608-14. doi: 10.1038/mp.2015.102. Epub 2015 Aug 4. PMID: 26239289; PMCID: PMC4740268.

[36] Zhang S, Zhornitsky S, Le TM, Li CR. Hypothalamic Responses to Cocaine and Food Cues in Individuals with Cocaine Dependence. Int J Neuropsychopharmacol. 2019 Dec 1;22(12):754-764. doi: 10.1093/ijnp/pyz044. PMID: 31420667; PMCID: PMC6929672.

[37] Jacobus J, Squeglia LM, Sorg SF, Nguyen-Louie TT, Tapert SF. Cortical thickness and neurocognition in adolescent marijuana and alcohol users following 28 days of monitored abstinence. J Stud Alcohol Drugs. 2014 Sep;75(5):729-43. doi: 10.15288/jsad.2014.75.729. PMID: 25208190; PMCID: PMC4161693.

[38] Stewart JL, May AC, Paulus MP. Bouncing back: Brain rehabilitation amid opioid and stimulant epidemics. Neuroimage Clin. 2019;24:102068. doi: 10.1016/j.nicl.2019.102068. Epub 2019 Nov 5. PMID: 31795056; PMCID: PMC6978215.

[39] Lim TV, Cardinal RN, Savulich G, Jones PS, Moustafa AA, Robbins TW, Ersche KD. Impairments in reinforcement learning do not explain enhanced habit formation in cocaine use disorder. Psychopharmacology (Berl). 2019 Aug;236(8):2359-2371. doi: 10.1007/s00213-019-05330-z. Epub 2019 Aug 1. PMID: 31372665; PMCID: PMC6695345.

[40] Mete M, Sakoglu U, Spence JS, Devous MD Sr, Harris TS, Adinoff B. Successful classification of cocaine dependence using brain imaging: a generalizable machine learning approach. BMC Bioinformatics. 2016 Oct 6;17(Suppl 13):357. doi: 10.1186/s12859-016-1218-z. PMID: 27766943; PMCID: PMC5073995.

[41] Cannella N, Cosa-Linan A, Takahashi T, Weber-Fahr W, Spanagel R. Cocaine addicted rats show reduced neural activity as revealed by manganese-enhanced MRI. Sci Rep. 2020 Nov 9;10(1):19353. doi: 10.1038/s41598-020-76182-3. PMID: 33168866; PMCID: PMC7653042.

[42] Pati S, Angel P, Drake RR, Wagner JJ, Cummings BS. Lipidomic changes in the rat hippocampus following cocaine conditioning,

extinction, and reinstatement of drug-seeking. Brain Behav. 2019 Dec;9(12):e01451. doi: 10.1002/brb3.1451. Epub 2019 Nov 7. PMID: 31701674; PMCID: PMC6908860.

[43] Li Z, Lei K, Coles CD, Lynch ME, Hu X. Longitudinal changes of amygdala functional connectivity in adolescents prenatally exposed to cocaine. Drug Alcohol Depend. 2019 Jul 1;200:50-58. doi: 10.1016/j.drugalcdep.2019.03.007. Epub 2019 Apr 30. PMID: 31085378; PMCID: PMC6607904.

[44] Karoly HC, Schacht JP, Jacobus J, Meredith LR, Taylor CT, Tapert SF, Gray KM, Squeglia LM. Preliminary evidence that computerized approach avoidance training is not associated with changes in fMRI cannabis cue reactivity in non-treatment-seeking adolescent cannabis users. Drug Alcohol Depend. 2019 Jul 1;200:145-152. doi: 10.1016/j.drugalcdep.2019.04.007. Epub 2019 May 14. PMID: 31132681; PMCID: PMC6635134.

[45] Shi J, Liu YL, Fang YX, Xu GZ, Zhai HF, Lu L. Traditional Chinese medicine in treatment of opiate addiction. Acta Pharmacol Sin. 2006 Oct;27(10):1303-8. doi: 10.1111/j.1745-7254. 2006.00431.x. PMID: 17007736.

[46] Zhou Y, Xiao S, Li C, Chen Z, Zhu C, Zhou Q, Ou J, Li J, Chen Y, Luo C, Mo Z. Extracellular Vesicle-Encapsulated miR-183-5p from Rhynchophylline-Treated H9c2 Cells Protect against Methamphetamine-Induced Dependence in Mouse Brain by Targeting NRG1. Evid Based Complement Alternat Med. 2021 Aug 26;2021:2136076. doi: 10.1155/2021/2136076. PMID: 34484386; PMCID: PMC8416368.